New Image For Women

Gerrie Pinckney and
Marge Swenson

Illustrated by Diana Dosh and Greg Bechtel

Reston Publishing Company, Inc.
A Prentice-Hall Company
Reston, Virginia

Because of the tremendous and widespread response to "New Image for Women," and "New Image for Men," many independent and professional organizations have adopted the texts as instructional material. Although we are very pleased by this enthusiastic response, the authors and the Fashion Academy Inc. cannot endorse any particular program of instruction with the exception of Fashion Academy Certified Consultants. This is not to imply that we do not recognize the quality of many other programs and hope that both books will continue to be of value to all who use them.

Before engaging professional assistance, however, we would urge the reader to consider the background and credibility of any fashion or color consultant just as one would in any other field.

CREDITS

Makeup by the Fashion Academy Inc.
Photography by Joel Swenson
Book design by L.J. Heart and Associates
Art Director: 'T' Hruska
Illustrations by Greg Bechtel and Diana Dosh
Hair styling by "Mr. Zachary's Hair Designs"
Eyeglasses by Lido Optical

2850 Mesa Verde Drive East
Costa Mesa, California 92626
(714) 979-8073

FASHION
ACADEMY INC.

Dedications

We dedicate this book to our husbands, George and Merrill, and to our children, for their love, support and sacrifice.

Much appreciation goes to our staff, Fashion Academy Certified Consultants, friends and students for their loyalty and encouragement.

FASHION
ACADEMY INC.

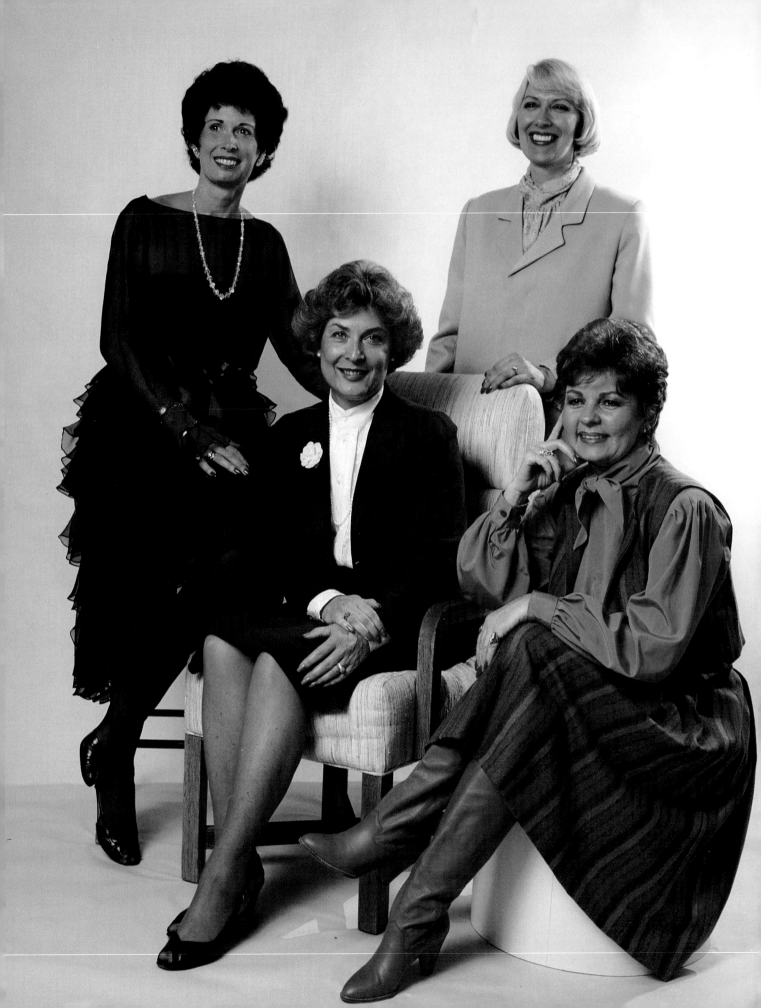

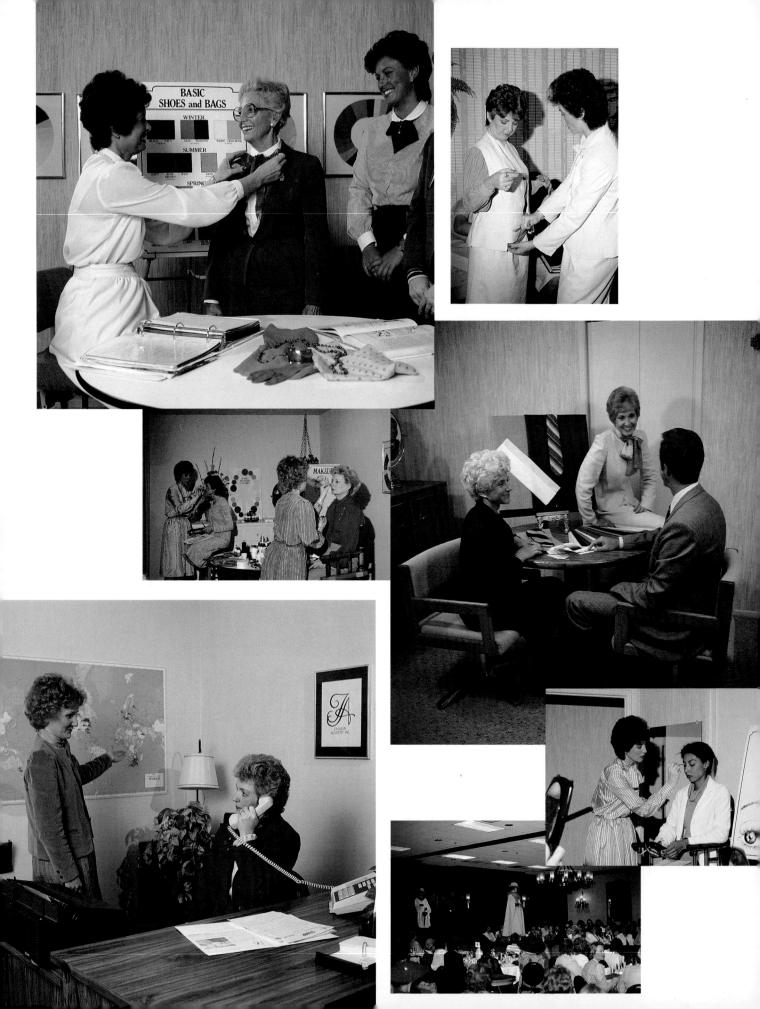

Since Eve selected her first fur for color and texture, then trimmed it to conform to body curves, women have been involved with fashion. To express no interest in how you cover your body is absurd. No one wears clothes simply to avoid being arrested or to keep warm. However, if you claim the latter, a blanket would do the job as well. Whether you accomplish the task of clothing your body with artistic efficiency or catch-as-catch-can, clothes represent a sizeable proportion of your budget. Because you are going to buy them anyway, why not become proficient enough to enjoy this aspect of your life?

While it may be vain and foolish to place too much importance on dress and grooming, it is downright foolhardy to pay too little attention to it. Research has provided irrefutable evidence that appearance does have impact on the way people judge you. Whether you like to admit it or not, you make a statement with your clothes and grooming.

Women go through cycles; the very young girl is striving to identify with her peer group. She often has no sense of identity. She strives to look like every other girl. It is not until she develops a degree of maturity and self-confidence that she is able to display any originality in her choice of clothing. The young married woman is often caught up with her home, small children and a low budget. Her figure and her wardrobe usually suffer. At 40, however, with her last child off her lap, she has more money and more time to devote to herself. If she has retained her figure or has the determination to get it back, she will experience a "fashion renaissance." Her efforts to achieve personal style, however, are often hampered by a confusing mumbo-jumbo of misinformation and advertising gimmicks. Many women give up because they lack knowledge of what is suitable for them at that age. Many more despair because they are unable to find suitable clothes for their figure. Manufacturers of ready-to-wear have shown a remarkable degree of ignorance and lack of sensitivity to the needs of the average woman, the one with the non-conforming body and a desire for lady-like, lasting, becoming clothes. The makers of clothing hope to brainwash us into wanting the newest bizarre style, regardless of how unsuitable it might be for our personalities, body types, budgets or lifestyles.

In an effort to simplify clothing selection, many texts on the topic have contributed to the difficulty by being too general. It is impossible to generalize about body types and personalities, let alone color or any other facet of an individual's total look. We have tried to be specific in describing the most common figure flaws and just as specific in offering solutions. Our aim has been to bring some organization to your method of clothing selection, to help you realize your potential in proper use of color and makeup techniques, to enlarge your horizons for possible hair styling and accessories and to help you gain an appreciation of yourself and your potential for beauty.

We have always taken a practical approach to wardrobe planning. The thousands of women who have taken our classes can't be bothered with complicated, time-consuming techniques of personal grooming or involved, expensive wardrobe plans. Their demand for simplicity has nothing to do with their degree of education, income or employment. The women we have taught have encompassed the total spectrum of age, race, profession and social strata. Women today are just too busy, whatever their position — they want their lives simplified and streamlined in the area of clothing and grooming, as well as everywhere else, but still want to amplify their own uniqueness.

Our total wardrobe planning and grooming concept has grown as a result of this need for a workable plan on the one hand, and on the other hand as a consequence of our actual involvement with creating fashion and observing the results on real, live functioning females with their figure flaws, weight problems and potential for beauty.

You will note that we urge purchase of classic, traditional styles for a basic wardrobe. We know that classics are smart investments. Fads, because they come and go, are expensive, but they can contribute spice in your life if chosen to conform with your age, body-type, personality and lifestyle.

It has been our function since 1960 to help women learn to use clothing more wisely — to look their absolute best with a minimum expenditure of money and time. In the years we have worked with women we have learned much and grown in appreciation of the uniqueness and delight of womanhood. We have watched our students become more attractive and self-confident, which enabled them to turn their thoughts outward, become more people-centered and develop charm — and that is our ultimate aim for you.

Marge and Gerrie
Fashion Academy
Costa Mesa, California

COLOR PALETTES

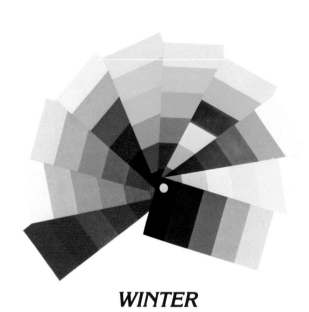

WINTER

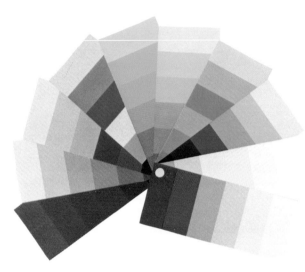

SUMMER

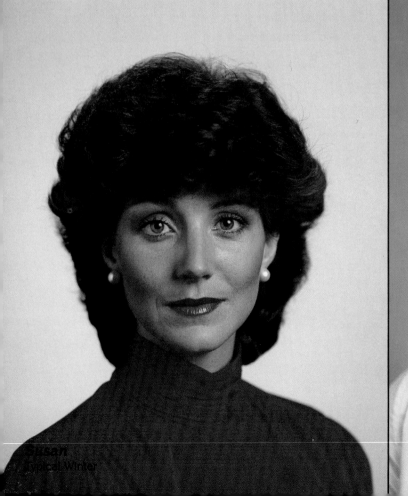

Susan
Typical Winter

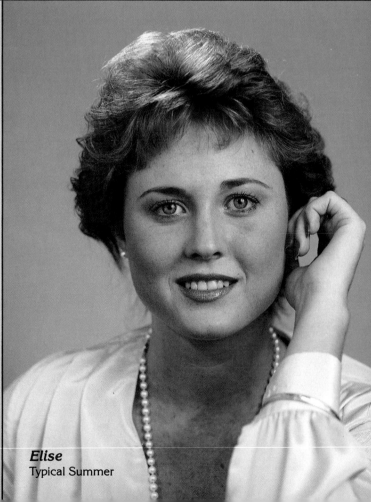

Elise
Typical Summer

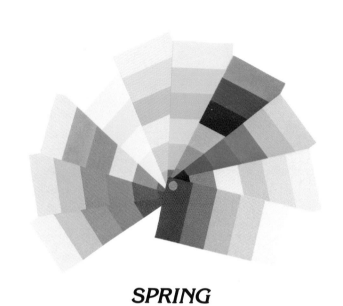

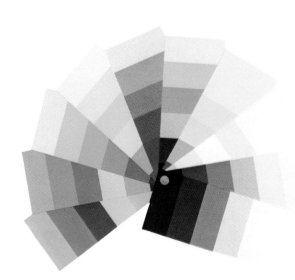

SPRING

AUTUMN

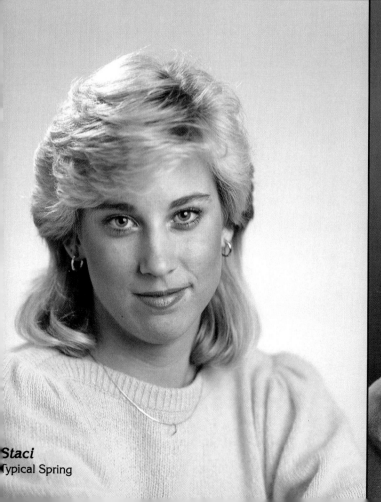

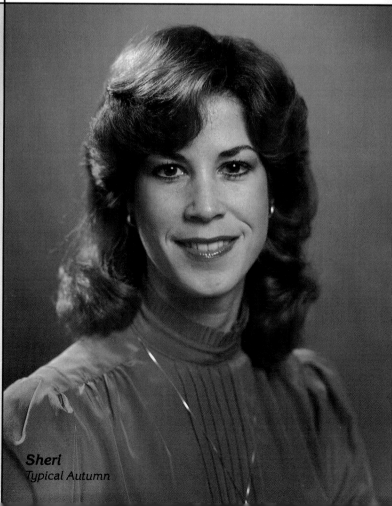

Staci
Typical Spring

Sheri
Typical Autumn

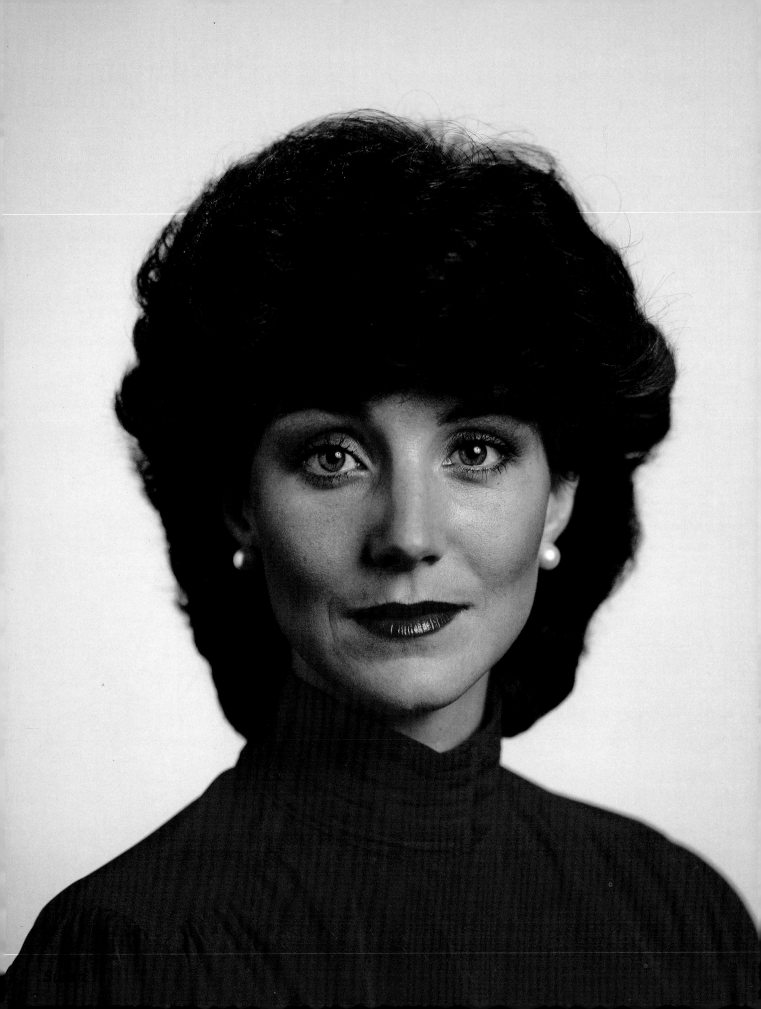

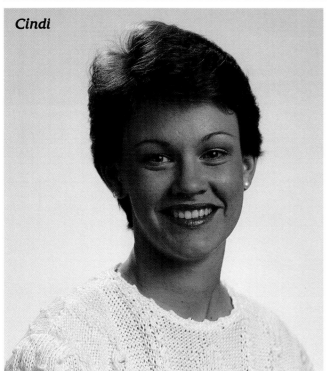

Cindi

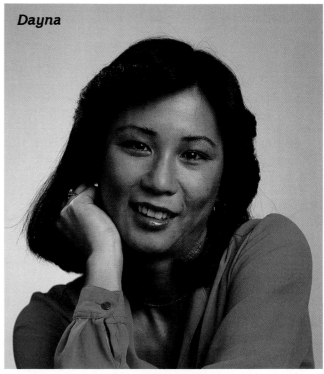

Dayna

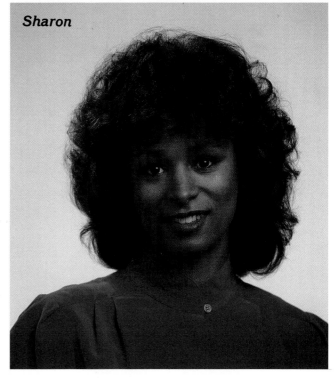

Sharon

WINTER SEASON

Susan: Light olive skin, gray-green eyes, dark brown hair

Cindi: Rose-beige skin, gray-blue eyes, medium brown hair

Dayna: Olive skin, brown-black eyes, black hair

Sharon: Brown skin, brown eyes, brown hair

The Winter woman wears the true basic primary colors. She also wears the true basic primary colors with blue added to them.

The Winter can wear all values of the primary colors from light to dark, but the intensity must be clear, not dusty.

Winter is the only season who wears black and chalk white successfully.

Winter and Summer are cousins because their colors are of a blue undertone. Some of their colors will overlap.

The key to the Winter color selection is: True or Blue and Clear. Winters wear silver jewelry which harmonizes with their skin and colors.

Use Of Color

NEUTRAL COLORS are chalk-white, true or blue grays, black, navy, gray-beiges. They are basic and will go any place, any time. Hair must be well groomed, makeup properly applied and you must be feeling well and have had adequate rest. A costume of all neutral colors is most elegant when harmonized with hair and eyes.

BASIC COLORS are the true or blue reds, blues and greens, medium to dark shades. They will go most any place, any time. They are very becoming because they add color to the face.

BRIGHT COLORS are more intense, medium to dark shades. They are used as bright accents with neutrals or mixed in prints. They are fun colors for active sportswear. If used solid in a large area, such as a dress, the fabric must be of good quality or it can look cheap. Bright colors make very sophisticated evening wear when made of a good fabric and simple design.

LIGHT COLORS are more feminine and delicate. They are good in lingerie, dressy blouses, scarves, summer wear and evening dresses with a fuller, more feminine design.

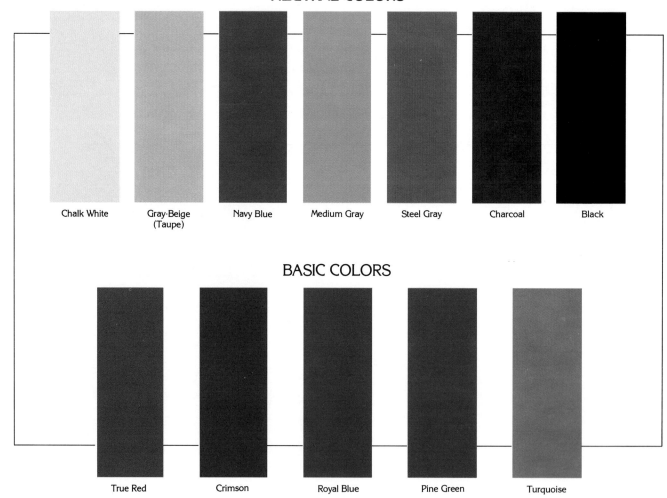

NEUTRAL COLORS

| Chalk White | Gray-Beige (Taupe) | Navy Blue | Medium Gray | Steel Gray | Charcoal | Black |

BASIC COLORS

| True Red | Crimson | Royal Blue | Pine Green | Turquoise |

BRIGHT COLORS

| Blue-Red | Lemon Yellow | True Green | True Blue | Royal Purple | Hot Pink |

| Fuchsia Magenta | Azalea Bright Maroon | Emerald Green | Turquoise | Hot Electric Blue | Periwinkle Blue |

LIGHT COLORS

| Ice Gray | Ice Green | Ice Yellow | Ice Pink | Ice Aqua | Ice Blue | Ice Violet | Ice Periwinkle |

13

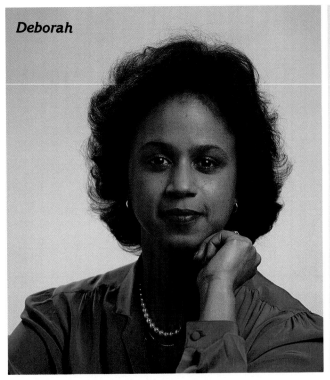

Deborah

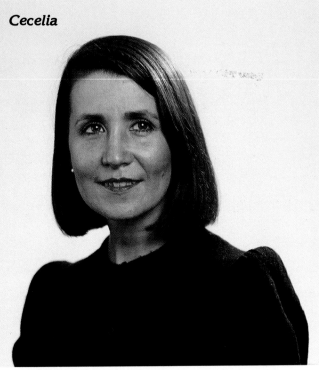

Cecelia

Deborah has brown skin, black-brown eyes, and black-brown hair; her appearance is typical of the American black race. Hers is a Classic-Romantic personality.

Cecelia has olive skin, gray-green-brown eyes and black-brown hair. Her Dramatic appearance is the product of her South American heritage.

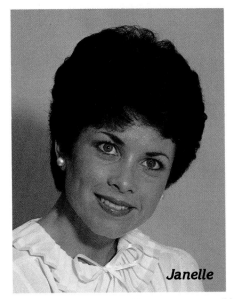

Janelle

There are more Winters in the world than any other season because there are more dark people. Due to mixed racial heritages, Winters can come from any nationality. Depending on heredity, their skin coloring can range from porcelain-white to rose-beige, light to dark olive, red-brown, yellow-brown, black-brown or blue-black. If Winters wear earthtones, in makeup or clothing, their skins can look sallow and lifeless.

Janelle has fair white skin, deep blue-gray eyes and black-brown hair. We call her a "Snow White" Winter. She typifies her Irish heritage.

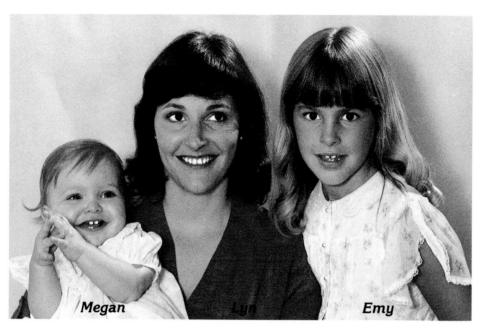

Megan   Lyn   Emy

Mother and daughters were all born with dark hair which then turned light ashy blonde, then golden honey. Both children will be dark like their mother when they are grown. Lyn, the mother, followed this typical Winter pattern.

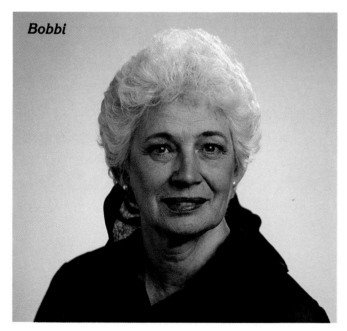

Bobbi

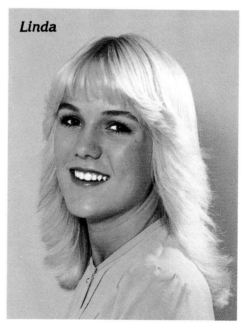

Linda

Bobbi has the beautiful silver-white hair typical of the mature, dark-haired Winter. She has rose-beige skin and grey-green eyes. Bobbi's hair was very dark brown as a young woman. If a completely grey-haired Winter dyes her hair dark, attempting to recapture the shade of her youth, it will be too harsh for her skin tone.

Linda, age 14, has beautiful olive skin which makes her appear tan all year round. Her striking blonde hair will grow gradually darker with maturity. Her eyes are deep gray-blue. Linda is not a typical Winter. Usually by age 14 the hair is much darker.

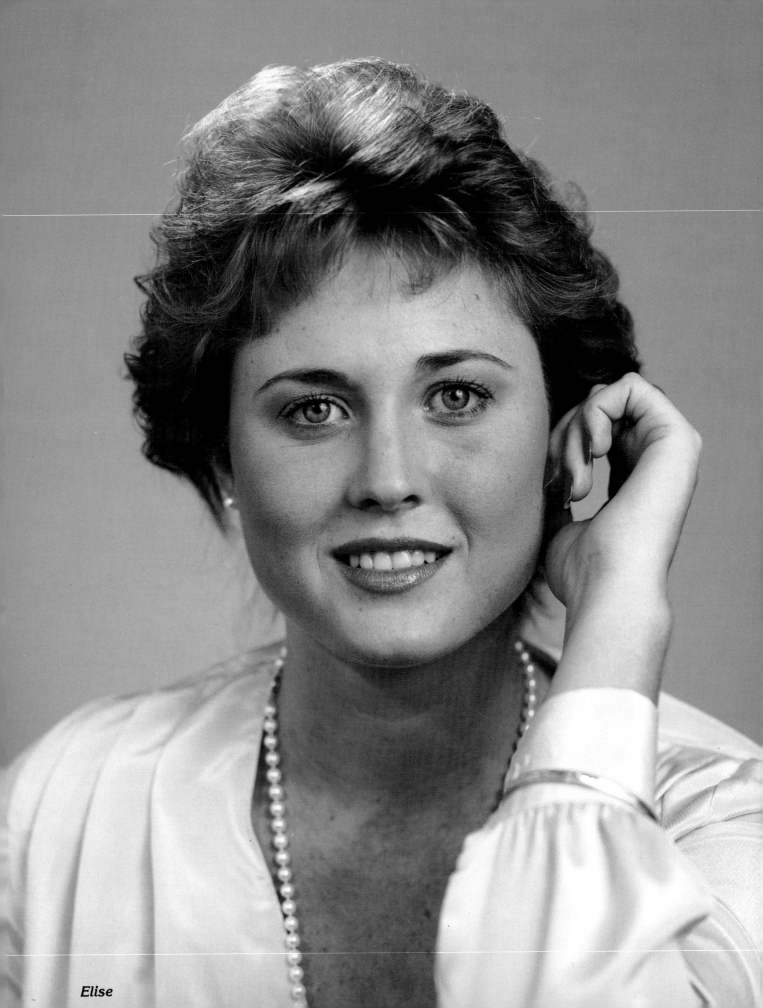

Elise

Ann

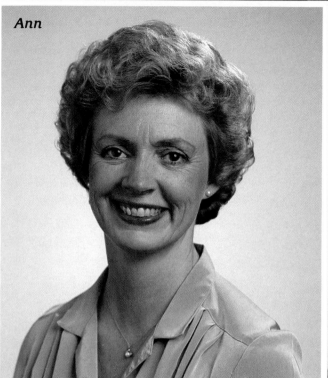

Mary Anne

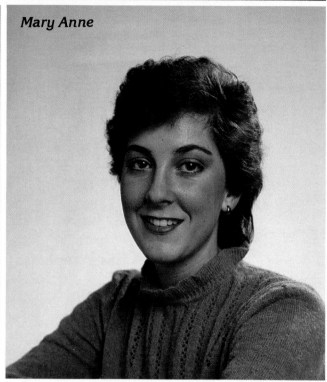

Carole

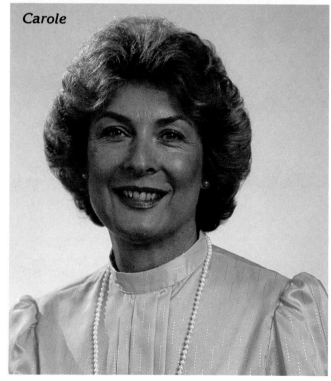

SUMMER SEASON

Elise: Rose pink skin, blue eyes, dark ash blonde hair

Ann: Fair pink skin, deep blue-gray eyes, light ash blonde hair

Mary Anne: Light rose beige skin, gray-green eyes, dark ash brown hair

Carole: Rose beige skin, blue-green (chameleon-like) eyes, light ash brown hair (highlighted)

The Summer woman wears dusty, muted shades of blue or rose undertones.

When colors are medium to light, they can be dusty or clear, but when they are from medium to dark, they should be dusty.

Dark, bright, intense colors will overpower the Summer person.

The key to Summer color selection is: Blue undertones of soft pastels to dusty dark tones.

Summer wears silver jewelry.

Use of Color

NEUTRAL COLORS are off-white, blue-gray, gray-navy, rose-beige and rose-brown. They are basic and will go any place, any time. Hair must be well groomed, makeup properly applied and you must be feeling well and have had adequate rest. A costume of all neutral colors is most elegant when harmonized with hair and eyes.

BASIC COLORS are the blue-reds, gray-blues and blue-greens, medium to dark shades. They will go most any place, any time. They are very becoming because they add color to the face.

BRIGHT COLORS are more intense, medium to dark shades. They are used as bright accents with neutrals or mixed in prints. They are fun colors for active sportswear. If used solid in a large area, such as a dress, the fabric must be of good quality or it can look cheap. Bright colors make very sophisticated evening wear when made of a good fabric and simple design.

LIGHT COLORS are more feminine and delicate. They are good in lingerie, dressy blouses, scarves, summer wear and evening dresses with a fuller, more feminine design.

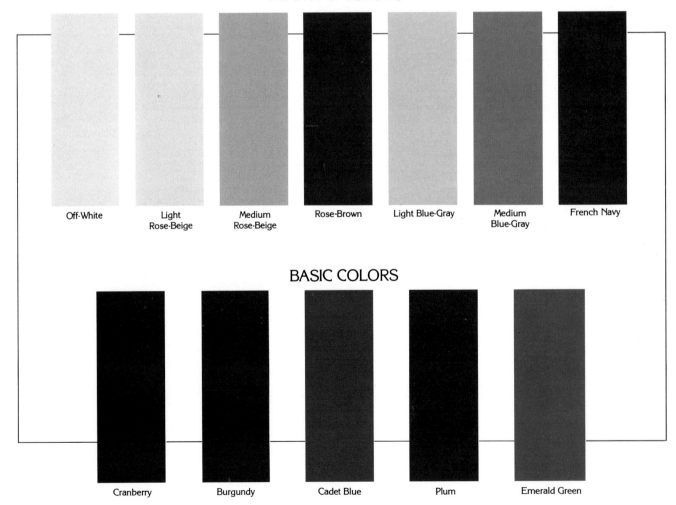

NEUTRAL COLORS

| Off-White | Light Rose-Beige | Medium Rose-Beige | Rose-Brown | Light Blue-Gray | Medium Blue-Gray | French Navy |

BASIC COLORS

| Cranberry | Burgundy | Cadet Blue | Plum | Emerald Green |

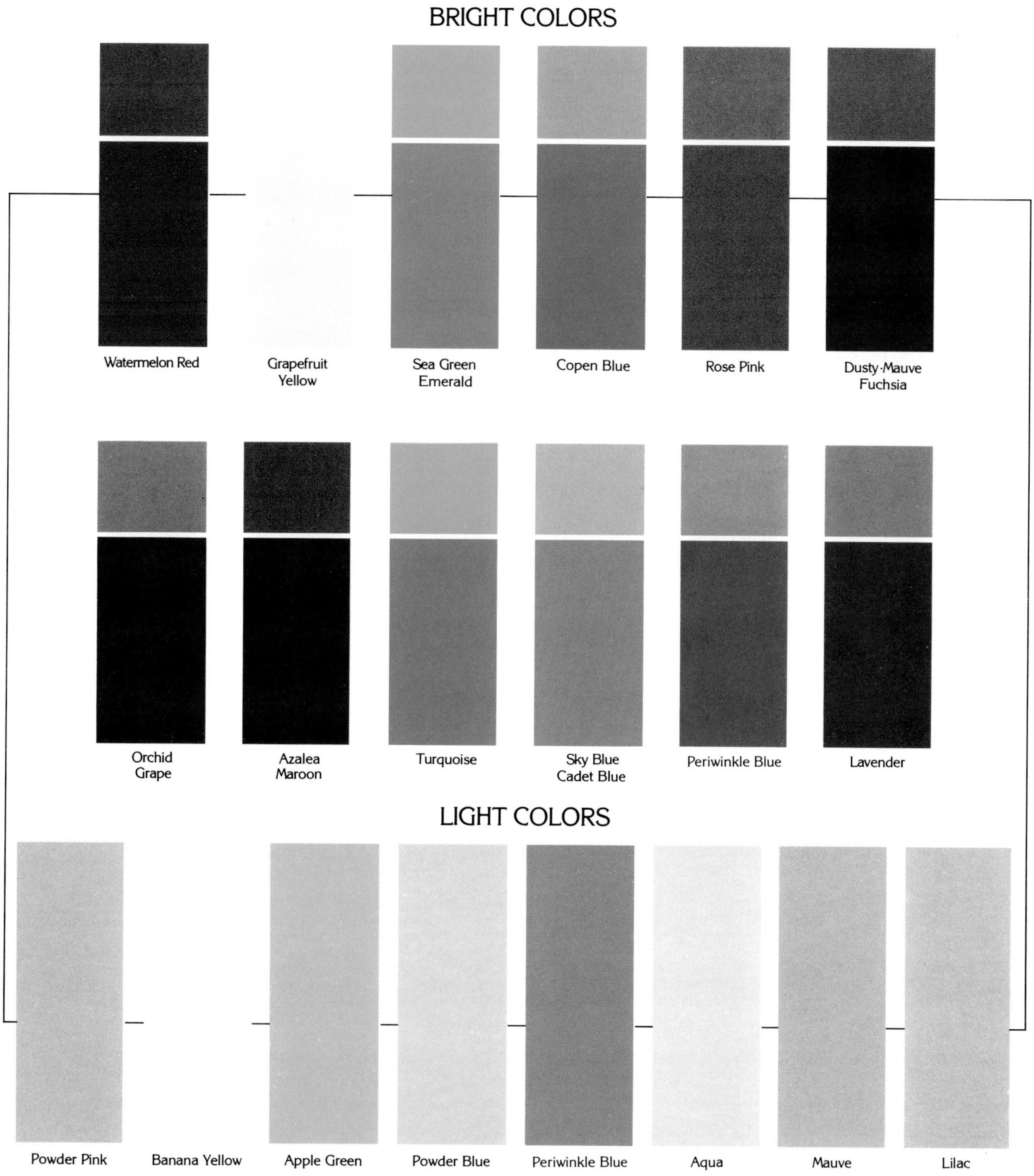

BRIGHT COLORS

Watermelon Red

Grapefruit
Yellow

Sea Green
Emerald

Copen Blue

Rose Pink

Dusty-Mauve
Fuchsia

Orchid
Grape

Azalea
Maroon

Turquoise

Sky Blue
Cadet Blue

Periwinkle Blue

Lavender

LIGHT COLORS

Powder Pink

Banana Yellow

Apple Green

Powder Blue

Periwinkle Blue

Aqua

Mauve

Lilac

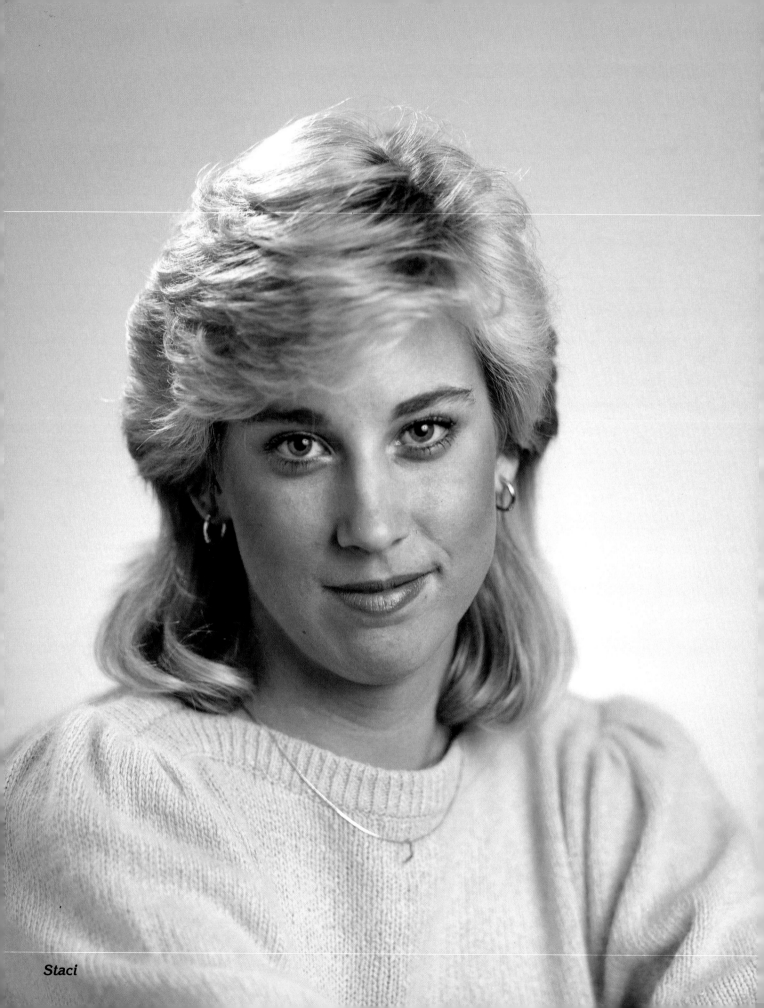

Staci

Terra

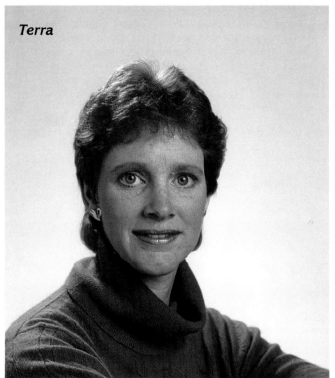

Linda

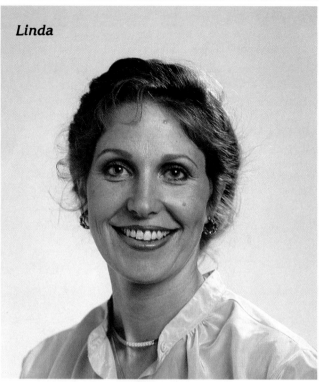

Anya

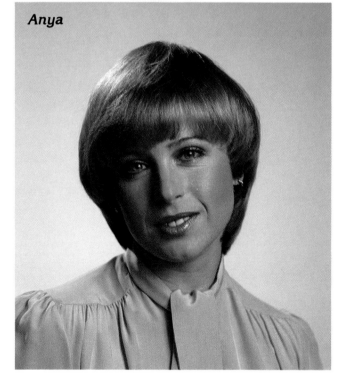

SPRING SEASON

Staci: The typical "Golden Girl." Warm peach skin, bright aqua eyes, golden blonde hair

Terra: Fair peach skin, bright blue eyes, bright red hair

Linda: Ivory skin, gray-blue eyes, light golden brown hair

Anya: Ivory skin, aqua eyes, light golden blonde hair

The Spring woman wears yellow undertones — warm, clear, fresh-fruit, spring bouquet colors.

Spring has the greatest range of colors of any season.

Her only limitation is that she cannot successfully wear clothes which are very dark.

The key to Spring color selection is: Yellow undertone, clear, medium to light colors.

Spring wears gold jewelry.

Use Of Color

NEUTRAL COLORS are warm white, warm grays, clear royal navy, warm golden beiges and golden-browns. They are basic and will go any place, any time. Hair must be well groomed, makeup properly applied and you must be feeling well and have had adequate rest. A costume of all neutral colors is most elegant when harmonized with hair and eyes.

BASIC COLORS are the clear yellow-reds, clear blues, clear yellow-greens, and clear golds in medium shades. They will go most any place, any time. They are very becoming because they add color to the face.

BRIGHT COLORS are more intense, medium to dark shades. They are used as bright accents with neutrals or mixed in prints. They are fun colors for active sportswear. If used solid in a large area, such as a dress, the fabric must be of good quality or it can look cheap. Bright colors make very sophisticated evening wear when made of a good fabric and simple design.

LIGHT COLORS are more feminine and delicate. They are good in lingerie, dressy blouses, scarves, summer wear and evening dresses with a fuller, more feminine design.

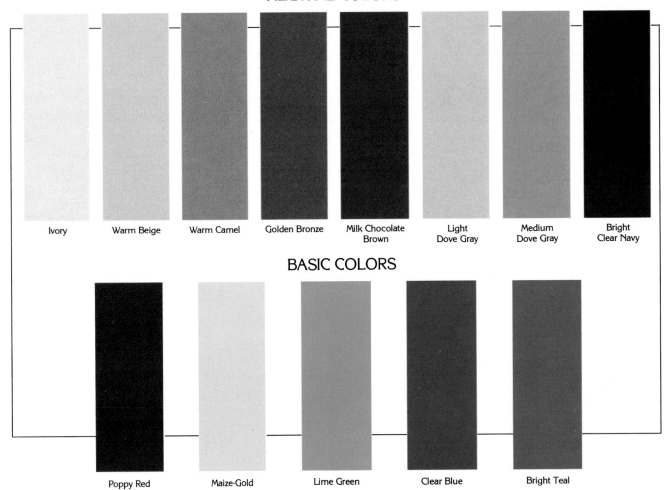

NEUTRAL COLORS

Ivory	Warm Beige	Warm Camel	Golden Bronze	Milk Chocolate Brown	Light Dove Gray	Medium Dove Gray	Bright Clear Navy

BASIC COLORS

Poppy Red	Maize-Gold	Lime Green	Clear Blue	Bright Teal

BRIGHT COLORS

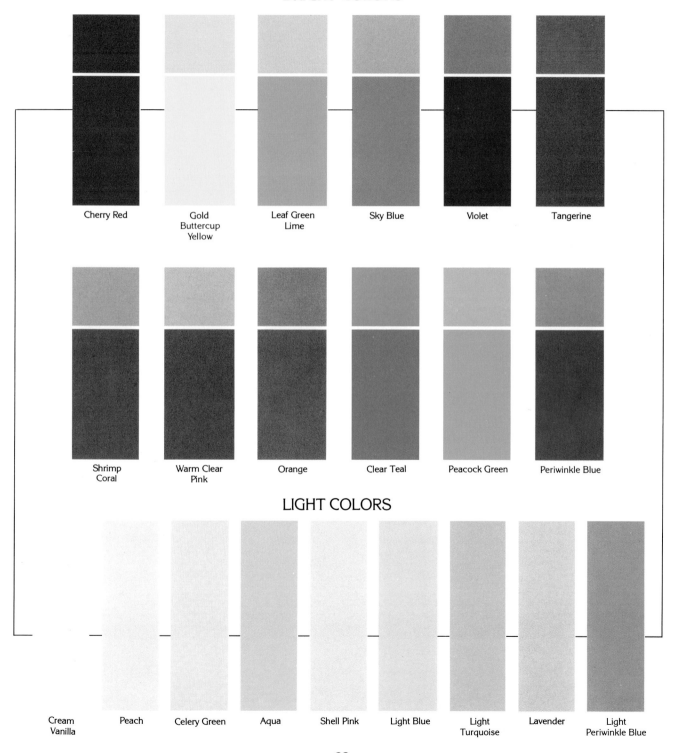

Cherry Red

Gold
Buttercup
Yellow

Leaf Green
Lime

Sky Blue

Violet

Tangerine

Shrimp
Coral

Warm Clear
Pink

Orange

Clear Teal

Peacock Green

Periwinkle Blue

LIGHT COLORS

Cream
Vanilla

Peach

Celery Green

Aqua

Shell Pink

Light Blue

Light
Turquoise

Lavender

Light
Periwinkle Blue

23

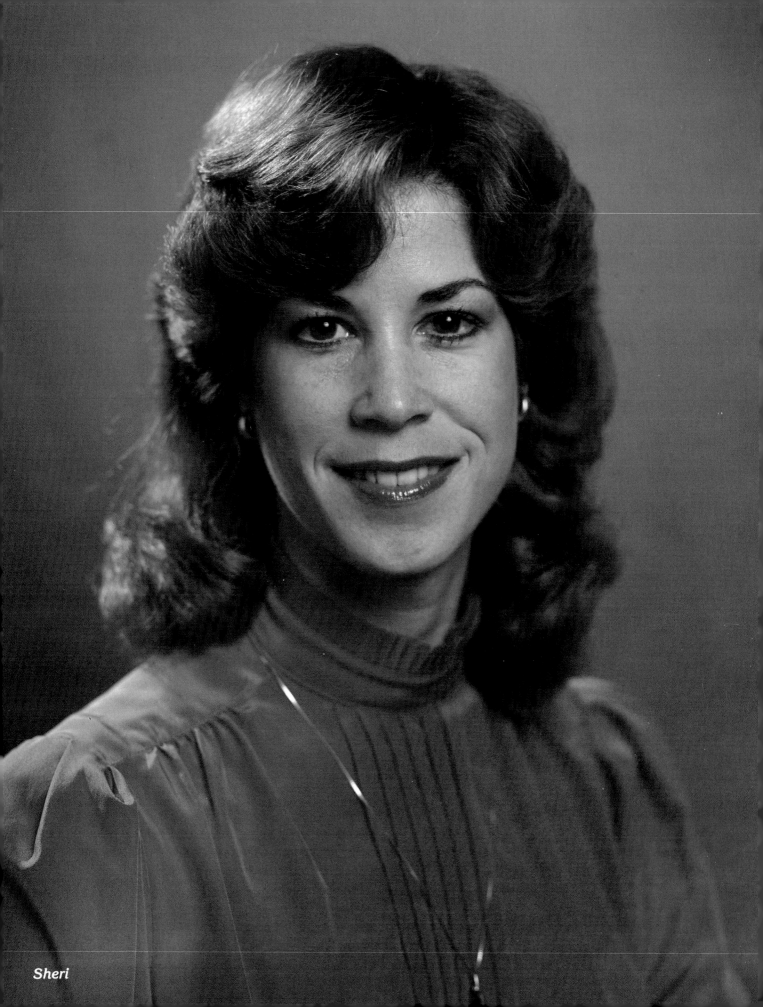

Sheri

Emelyn

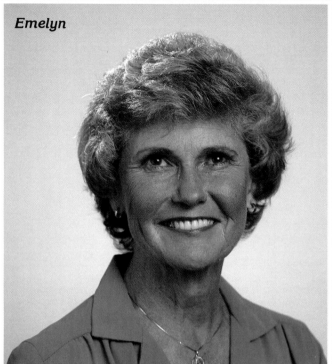

Carolyn

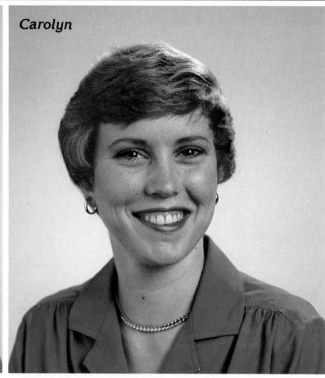

Sondra

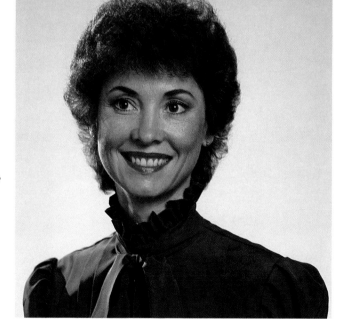

AUTUMN SEASON

Sheri: Peach beige skin, golden brown eyes, medium brown hair with gold highlights

Emelyn: Light peach skin, brown eyes, medium brown hair turning warm gray

Carolyn: Light beige skin, amber brown eyes, medium warm brown hair

Sondra: Fair warm ivory skin, olive brown eyes, dark chestnut brown hair

The Autumn woman wears yellow undertones, earthy muted shades and colors of metal and wood.

Spring and Autumn are cousins. A few of their warm, clear colors will overlap, especially in yellows, oranges and browns.

The key to Autumn color selection is: Yellow undertone, dusty, muted, earth tones.

Autumn wears gold jewelry.

Use Of Color

NEUTRAL COLORS are warm white, warm beige and warm brown. They are basic and will go any place, any time. Hair must be well groomed, makeup properly applied and you must be feeling well and have had adequate rest. A costume of neutral colors is most elegant when harmonized with hair and eyes.

BASIC COLORS are the yellow-reds, teal blues, yellow-greens and golds, medium to dark shades. They will go most any place, any time. They are very becoming because they add color to the face.

BRIGHT COLORS are more intense, medium to dark shades. They are used as bright accents with neutrals or mixed in prints. They are fun colors for active sportswear. If used solid in a large area, such as a dress, the fabric must be of good quality or it can look cheap. Bright colors make very sophisticated evening wear when made of a good fabric and simple design.

LIGHT COLORS are more feminine and delicate. They are good in lingerie, dressy blouses, scarves, summer wear and evening dresses with a fuller, more feminine design.

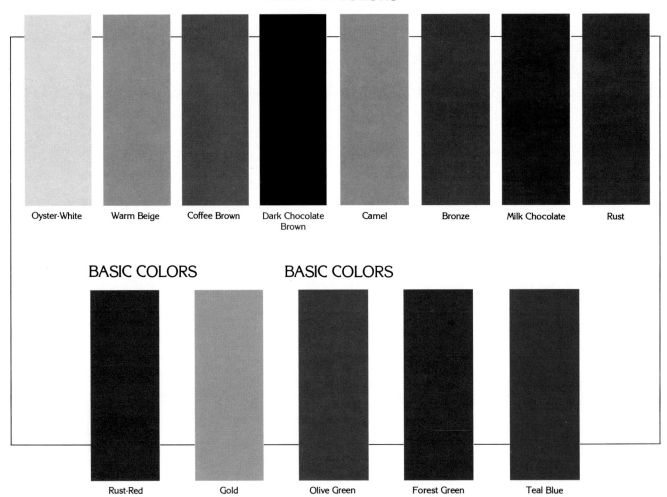

NEUTRAL COLORS

| Oyster-White | Warm Beige | Coffee Brown | Dark Chocolate Brown | Camel | Bronze | Milk Chocolate | Rust |

BASIC COLORS   BASIC COLORS

| Rust-Red | Gold | Olive Green | Forest Green | Teal Blue |

BRIGHT COLORS

Brick Red Flame	Pumpkin Sun Yellow	Lime Green Kelly	Teal Blue	Gold Mustard	Orange

Terra-Cotta Rust	Turquoise	Carrot Tangerine	Avocado Moss Green	Sage Jade	Periwinkle Blue

LIGHT COLORS

LIGHT COLORS

Cream-Vanilla	Apricot	Light Gold	Light Sage Green	Aqua	Peach	Light Turquoise	Periwinkle Blue

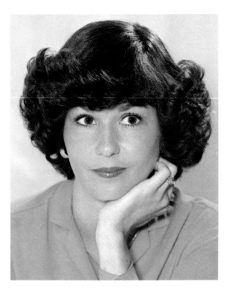

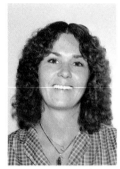

Wendy

Before

After

Wendy is a beautiful Romantic-Natural Winter, masquerading as a Natural Autumn.

After

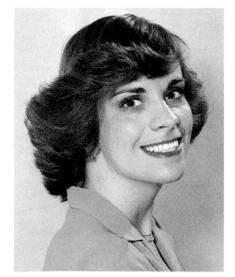

Naomi

Before

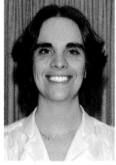

Naomi needed her brows shaped to enhance her big, beautiful eyes. A good hair style and proper makeup revealed a beautiful Natural-Classic Winter Woman with a charming, friendly personality.

April, an adorable Spring Gamin with a bubbly personality, needed a smoother style to bring out the beauty of her blonde hair.

April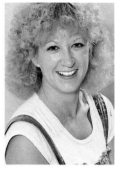

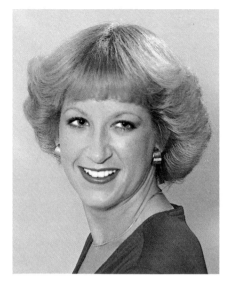

Before   **After**

Lisa

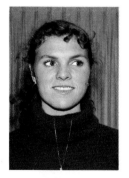

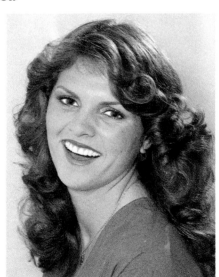

Before

Lisa is a 19-year-old Autumn Natural-Romantic. She has a round face, large eyes and naturally curly hair. Bulky turtlenecks and pulled-back hair emphasize her only negative. Soft, feathered curls enhance her Romantic appeal.

After

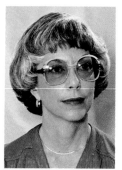

Roselyn

Before

Roselyn, a Classic Winter. Frames too light — lenses too dark.

After

Rimless glasses look better with gray hair and classic feminine features.

Suzan

Suzan, a Classic Winter. Frames too large and droopy — wrong color.

After

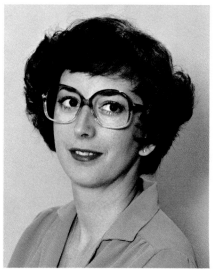

Before

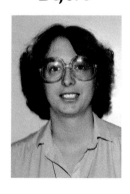

Frames give a lift to her face and harmonize with hair color

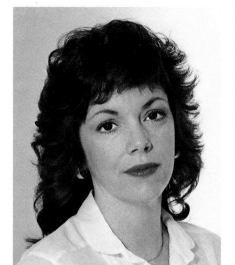

Sue

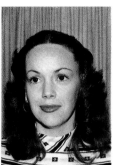

Before

After

Sue's long face and high forehead needed a soft bang. Using the correct Winter makeup brings out her Romantic feminine beauty.

After

Joie is a Winter doll! Wearing her fine, limp hair long failed to emphasize her animated Gamin features and large, beautiful eyes.

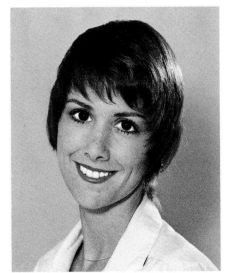

Before

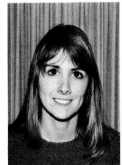

Joie

31

Five Basic Primary Colors

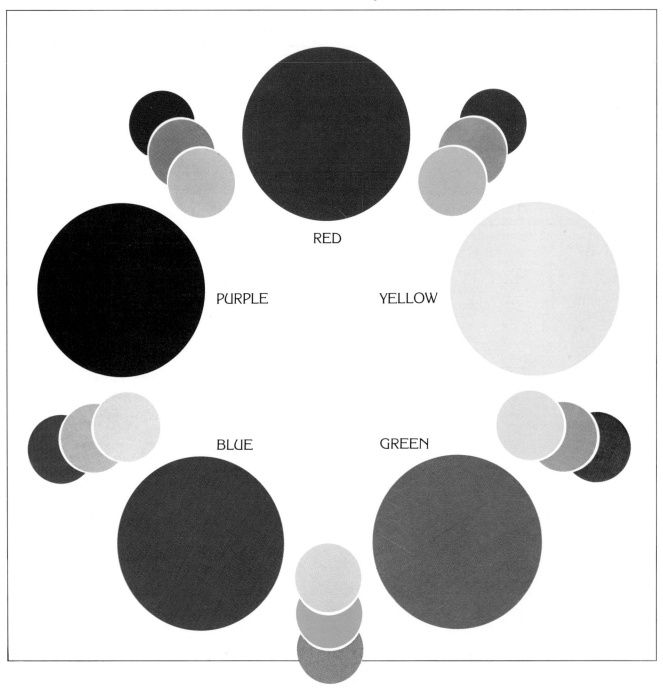

RED

PURPLE   YELLOW

BLUE   GREEN

*Combination of primary colors
are shown between primaries.*

Munsell Color Theory

At the Fashion Academy we have based our color concept on a color theory established by Albert H. Munsell, the greatest American colorist. Munsell's work is classical. It established permanent values in the art and science of color. His theory is considered the most logical and understandable in existence. Accepted by the U.S. Department of Agriculture and the *Encyclopedia Britannica*, it is used by most artists, dress designers, interior decorators and architects.

Munsell's theory is based on five *basic primary colors: red, yellow, green, blue and purple.* Munsell eliminated orange from his primary palette because he felt the inclusion of orange resulted in an unbalanced color wheel with too much yellow. We agree, because we have also found that yellow is the least becoming color on most people. You will note that we have eliminated orange from the Winter and Summer palettes. From Munsell's five basic hues are produced all the intermediate colors. Your selection of becoming colors is almost unlimited as long as you remember a few basic rules: *Everyone can wear all five of the basic primary colors depending on the undertone, the value and the clarity of a color.*

Before we go on to discuss the role of color in fashion, let us define a few terms:

Hue means color. It is the quality which distinguishes one color from another — for example, red from blue.

Undertone describes the color you get when you take the five basic hues and add either blue or yellow to them. For example, undertones can be a blue-red or a yellow-red, a blue-green or a yellow-green.

Value is the quality of lightness or darkness found in a color. It differentiates a light blue from a dark blue, for example, or a light pink from a maroon.

Clarity or *Chroma* is the quality of brightness or dullness of a color. Compare a fresh new leaf, strong and bright in color, to the same leaf in the autumn — dull and dusty. Contrast a clear pink to a muted dusty pink.

Winters wear the true basic primary hues and the five hues with blue added to them. Winter colors, whether true or blue, are clear. You can wear all of your colors in values from icy light to almost black.

Summers wear the five basic primary hues with blue added to them. Their colors are most becoming when they are muted or dusty. You can wear medium to light values of your colors whether clear or muted, but any hue which is medium to dark in value must be muted.

Springs wear the five basic primary hues with yellow added. Their colors are clear. Springs look best in shades which are medium to light in value. The darker colors are too strong for their coloring. Your coats and suits may be closer to Autumn because woolen fabrics often appear to be muted. Just be certain your blouses and scarves are in your clear shades.

Autumns wear the five primary hues with yellow added and they are muted or dusty. Many of Autumn's colors overlap with Spring, especially in the browns and golds. It is much easier for an Autumn to borrow the clear colors of Spring than for Spring to borrow the dusty shades of Autumn. The Autumn woman can successfully borrow Spring's yellow undertoned hues which are clear and *bright*, but not those which are clear and *light*. You should also avoid the blues and pinks of the Spring palette.

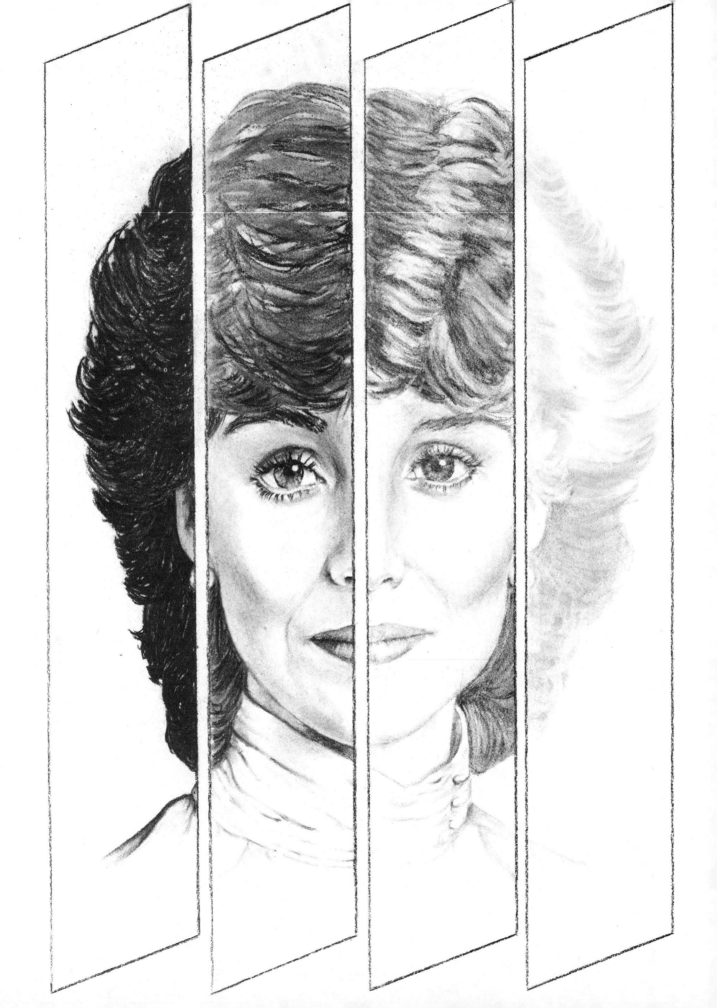

CHAPTER ONE

The Shades Of You

YOUR COLOR PALETTE

There are four factors involved in any garment or costume you might wear: color, line, personality and lifestyle. While these four are all important, color is by far the most intriguing and the first thing people see. Because color sets the stage, we will discuss color first.

Color Is The Key

You choose your clothing, your makeup, your accessories, your home decor, and sometimes even your car according to your taste in color. If left entirely alone, it is possible that by nature you would choose to wear the colors which are best for you. However, you may have been sidetracked through the influence of others: your mother, friends, fashion, fads, or what has been available in the stores. If you take a pre-school-age child shopping, nine times out of ten she will know what is best for her in terms of color, line and personality. Once she starts school, however, the test will not work because she is then influenced by her peer group.

We wish there were a magic method for you to determine your best colors. Most of you need no magic, however, because you will instinctively gravitate toward the garments most flattering to you. Those who may not have a good eye for color or an objective attitude because of preconceived notions might ask for help from friends or family.

At this point let's separate clothing choice from home decorating.

The colors you wear are not part of your environment. Once you put them on your back you do not see yourself. Colors in a room, however, influence us mentally, physically and emotionally. The majority of people will decorate in earth tones because these colors are warm inviting and cozy. But just because you can live contentedly surrounded by earth tones does not necessarily mean you should wear them. The reverse is also true; many people who look best in the cooler colors could not decorate in those colors because they would freeze to death.

In decorating, you must consider the personalities of those living in the home, the exposure of the room, and the feeling you wish to achieve. You may look terrific in rust, but you may not be able to stand living with it. Gray could be your best color to wear, but you wouldn't necessarily want a gray house.

Colors are usually divided into two undertones: yellow or blue. We have found that those who wear the yellow undertones most successfully are usually high-key people and may enjoy cooler tones in their environment to calm them down. Conversely, the people who wear the blue undertones well tend to be more low-key and enjoy warm undertones in their homes to give them a lift.

The Seasons Of Color

We have adapted the seasonal names Winter, Summer, Spring and Autumn into a total wardrobe planning concept because the colors fall naturally into these groupings — and it is much more fun to be a Spring, for example, than a Number Three.

The seasons are divided first into two groups: Winter and Summer with a blue undertone, and Spring and Autumn with a yellow undertone.

The colors are then divided again according to clarity. Winter and Spring are clear, and Summer and Autumn are dusty.

The main message of this book is that you can wear any color you wish and look all right, but why should you look just all right when you could look smashing in colors from your own color palette?

We have really not taken anything away from you — there are only five hues, and you can wear them all. We are merely guiding you into the proper grouping that will harmonize best with your skin, eyes and hair. You will discover colors in your palette you have never thought of wearing.

We are not trying to change you into something that you are not. We are trying to guide you to the place where Mother Nature intended you to be. We have found that Mother Nature knew what she was doing. We have never seen a woman whose eyes, skin and hair did not go well together, but we do see constantly women who try to change the combination around. What they end up with is a poor imitation of the real thing. Some people have excellent coloring and don't look bad in most colors, but others can't cheat; they can't get away with wearing just any color. Have you ever had someone ask, "Don't you feel well today?" You think, "I felt fine when I got up," but a few comments like that throughout the day and by evening you are wondering if perhaps you don't feel too well! Your outfit could be beautiful, but what is it doing for you?

It is difficult to categorize people by their appearance. They look at each other and say, "How can we all be the same season? We don't even look alike!" What you have to keep in mind is that there are varied shades of skin, eyes and

hair within any one season.

Basically, all those in the same season have the same undertone of skin and will look best in the same undertone of colors.

That is the key — undertone of the skin!

We realize that there are some people who can wear colors from other seasons and look O.K. But you cannot plan a wardrobe that way, by combining colors from both undertones. That is why people come to us. They have a closet full of clothes and nothing to wear.

We must give you the discipline of a season to help you have a well-planned and coordinated wardrobe.

This concept gives you a palette of colors — all of which will be becoming, all of which coordinate.

There is no one who can wear colors from both undertones and of all values and intensities and look equally good in them all.

It is very difficult for you to see yourself objectively. We all have preconceived ideas of what we look like or how we would like to look. Did you ever have a dress or an outfit in which you felt beautiful? We have found that if you will think back to those colors in which you have felt the best and in which you may have received the most compliments, you might have a good clue as to which colors are best for you.

What Determines Your Season?

Your season is determined by your skin, your eyes and your hair. Skin is the most important. Next, eyes and hair. Your season cannot be determined by just one of these three, especially the eyes, because there are so many variations of eye color from one season to another. We must consider all three in the final analysis. Mother Nature coordinated all three to go together and she knew what she was doing.

SKIN — Just as we find cool and warm undertones in colors, we find cool and warm undertones in skin. All skin has a blue undertone with a purple base, or it has a yellow undertone with a green base. The basic undertone does not change although it may fade with age. You may tan or freckle, but people tan different shades depending on skin tone. Some people have good natural coloring, others are sallow. Wearing the right colors will make blemishes appear to fade, make wrinkles less noticeable and enhance the natural skin tone. Various conditions can affect the outward appearance of the skin: illness, fatigue, diet (carrots and acidic foods and juices), use of tobacco or alcohol, extreme suntan, hair dyed the wrong color and use of the wrong color of makeup.

Those women who do not have good coloring (natural rosy cheeks) need the help of the right makeup to look really good, even in their own colors.

EYES — Eye color usually changes from birth to childhood, and again in maturity. The normal pattern is that you are born with dark blue eyes, which then change to a color which later fades with age. Your eyes are usually darker, brighter and more clear in youth than they are in maturity. We have found that blue-eyed people have more pink in their skin and brown-eyed people tend to be more sallow.

HAIR — Hair complements your skin tone. It may have as many as seven different shades. Hair color changes with age. You may have been born with dark hair; then it turned blonde, later it went medium or dark and then turned gray. Some women's hair color changes weekly. What we are trying to create is a harmony between skin, eyes, hair and clothing. If you dye your hair, you must choose a color on the chart which is one or two shades lighter than your natural color or it will be too dark.

Self-Discovery

Our exercise in self-discovery can be an exciting experience. It will require objectivity, honesty and a good memory of your childhood coloring, unhampered by your mother's imaginings. We are interested in the *real you*. Keep in mind your skin coloring without makeup or a tan, your eye color as a child and adult, your hair color as a child, as a young woman and your *true* hair color as an adult. This could be a little difficult for those of you who have not seen your natural hair color for a long time.

Read the descriptions of all four seasons. Which coloring and inner season most nearly describe you and which group of colors have you most enjoyed wearing?

The Winter Woman

There are more Winters in the world than any other season because there are more dark people. Because of mixed racial heritages, Winters can come from any nationality. Southern European and South American people are usually Winters with light to dark olive skin. The dark Irish and Welsh are often Winters with their striking contrast of light skin and dark hair. American Indians are Winters with dark red-brown or yellow-brown skin. No doubt it was the red-brown shade of skin which led to Indians being called "redskins." The Polynesians and people of Eastern Asia and India are Winters with skin ranging from olive-brown to black.

Orientals are all Winters. Depending on their heredity, their skin coloring can range from porcelain white to dark yellow-brown.

The Winter season takes in all Blacks, even though they may be of different shades depending on their heredity. The very dark blue Black woman can probably wear any season's colors, but we put her in the Winter season because she looks best in its clear, strong colors, and the emphasis on her best season gives her discipline in wardrobe planning. The light to dark brown Blacks should never wear the warm, muted Autumn shades because those colors turn their skins sallow.

The darker the skin, as with Blacks, the more noticeable the blue undertone. The yellow overcast is more noticeable in the brown-skinned people. This yellow cast makes them appear sallow.

Most Winters tan easily. Some don't tan at all. Others freckle. This is due to the red pigment of their skin. The tan of a Winter is usually a reddish brown tan and can look dirty if she gets too dark.

WINTER SKIN — Winters have a blue undertone with a purple base in their skin. Light to dark olive is the most common of the Winter skin tones, but it is also the hardest in which to detect the blue undertone because the skin is usually thicker, causing it to look yellow. The blue undertone of the skin, influenced by the yellow overtone, produces a grayish cast. This is especially noticeable when the olive-skinned person is tired or ill. Do not confuse olive skin with yellow-beige skin which has a green base, as found in the Autumn-Spring people. If you put yellow-undertoned colors on olive skin, that skin will look very yellow, sallow and tired. By putting blue-undertoned colors on olive skin, you will bring out the purple base, making the skin look more rosy, healthy and alive.

Winters are prone to dark circles under the eyes. Due to the purple base, their eyelids and lips take on a blue-red cast. Winters with dark lips have trouble with lipstick turning very dark. They can go without lipstick better than other seasons and not look too washed out.

WINTER EYES — All eye colors can be found in the Winter season, but brown is predominant. Brown eyes might range from a very light, golden-brown to a medium olive-brown, to a dark brown, to a black-brown. Often in the brown-eyed Winter you will see a violet tint around the pupil and a gray ring around the iris. You may see gold and/or green flecks in the light to medium brown eyes. Blue eyes found in Winters usually have gray in them. Some blue eyes have light flecks in them which look like granite or slate. When the eye is blue you will generally find more pink in the skin. Green eyes found in Winter are usually a clear gray-green or green with gold flecks. These green eyes often have a gray ring around the iris. Turquoise eyes, a blue-green combination often with a grayish cast, are found in Winter. Winter hazel eyes have a combination of blue, green and brown, with the blue or green more toward the outside of the iris and the brown stronger near the pupil. Some Winters have eyes resembling a German brown trout with dark brown-black and gold flecks.

Infrequent combinations found in Winter are eyes resembling a light blue or green transparent marble and a deep royal blue eye with a violet ring around the pupil shading into the blue iris, which gives the impression of being a violet eye. The eye can look blue or violet, depending on the colors worn or the mood of the person.

Those who have from light to deep rose-beige skin usually will have a blue or gray shade in their eye. Brown or hazel-eyed Winters are usually more sallow, which would indicate that less blue is coming through in the skin. This could trick you into thinking that you are a yellow-beige-skinned Autumn.

Winter Skin Tones:
  White
  Light to deep rose-beige
  Light to dark olive
  Black
  Brown-black
  Brown

Winter Eyes Are:
  Light to dark brown
  Black-brown
  Blue-gray
  Gray-green
  Yellow-green
  Turquoise
  Dark blue-violet
  Hazel

WINTER HAIR — Winters may have been towheads as children, others golden honey blonde, turning dark with maturity. They rarely stay blonde as adults. Winters will often gray prematurely. The darker the hair, the more gracefully it grays. When Winters turn gray, it is a silver-gray. Through the effects of exposure to the sun, hair sprays, shampoos or excessive smoking, their hair may acquire a yellow tinge. Winters should protect their hair from the sun. Light to medium to dark brown Winter hair will have a cool quality to the hair. Young people with cool brown hair might appear to have warm brown hair because of overexposure to the sun which has bleached the ends. The true hair color can be determined at the roots on the back of the head near the neck. This same type of hair will often turn very dark with maturity when it is no longer exposed to so much sunlight.

Winters with dark brown hair will typically turn quite dark just before turning gray.

Many Winters have chestnut brown hair which has red highlights in it, especially in warmer climates where the hair is exposed to sun bleaching. Those natural red highlights are more of a copper-red than an orange-red. This type of Winter often dyes her hair red, but not being a true redhead, she will look hard and sallow, especially as she matures. This is the Winter that gets sidetracked into wearing Autumn colors to match her hair. An olive-skinned Winter who has dyed red hair will often look as if her face is dirty. A Winter who dyes her hair blonde, red or black will have a hard, cheap look. Winters should never frost their hair. Frosted hair rushes the graying process before the skin and eyes are ready for it, and it is aging. Winter hair which has been frosted has a tendency to take on a yellow cast.

Winter Hair Is:
Platinum blonde, golden-brown (on young girls)
Medium to dark brown
Chestnut brown
Black-brown or black
Gray (silver)

YOUR INNER SEASON — Over the years, we have noticed similarities between people of the same season in the way they act and look at life. We make no assertion that our conclusions are scientific. Our comments on the "inner season" are all in fun — but they can be uncanny in accuracy. The inner season has nothing to do with astrology; it is nothing mysterious or mystical. The comments are based solely on our pleasant association with and observations of students.

The Winter woman stands out in a crowd because of her definite coloring and strong personality. The combination of vivid coloring and her air of self-assurance may make her appear aloof. Possessing a will of iron, she is sometimes stubborn, domineering or aggressive; she may have a sharp tongue. She uses a positive approach and retains her composure in a crisis. The Winter woman is decisive and rarely impulsive, a strong leader who can delegate authority. If she is not completely sure of herself in any situation she manages to project a self-assured facade.

She has few intimate friends, but is admired and respected by her peers. An early riser, she is ambitious, hard-working and intelligently organized. Winter makes a good career woman. She loves to make long-range plans with every detail written down. She makes notes to herself to help organize her thoughts and plan her day, but sometimes she is so over-organized that her accomplishments do not compare with her long lists. The Winter woman makes a great friend if you can ever get really well-acquainted with one. When you get to know her, she is fun and relaxing to be with, but don't ever betray her confidence; she never forgets. She could be compared to a diamond — sparkling, expensive and sharp on the edges.

It is important for Winters to understand the effect they have on other people. Their darkness makes them less approachable; therefore, Winters usually must make the overtures of friendship, be the first to smile and extend a cordial greeting. The Winter woman must be particularly supportive of acquaintances, friends and especially of employees over whom she might have authority. Her positive approach, decisiveness and strong leadership can be frightening, especially if she is aggressive.

A Winter's path through life will be smoother if she can learn to soften her approach. She must recognize that by just standing there she can intimidate other people.

The Summer Woman

Some of the most beautiful women in the world are Summers. Their rosy, delicate coloring and classic reserve epitomize femininity. The Summer season combines a racial mixture. Many are found with a heritage from the British Isles, the Scandinavian countries, the Netherlands and Northern European countries. We have found fewer Summers in our classes. We do not necessarily feel that there are fewer Summers among the population, but we do attest to the fact that a Summer is less inclined to spend time or money for this type of course for herself. She would freely give it to her daughter, however. If we can once convince a Summer that she can develop her full potential by utilizing the things we teach, she becomes our most devoted fan and talkative convert.

An interesting note: We have found in our travels around the country that many other color consultants, due perhaps to a poor color eye or lack of training, put many people who are not Summers into this season.

SUMMER SKIN — Summer skin has a blue undertone which gives it a pink, rosy cast. The blue undertone is usually easier to see in the Summer than it is in the Winter woman.

Fair Summers have a delicate, cameo look. Summers seem to have thin skins. They often flush easily. When they blush, the color is instant. Summers with deeper rose-beige skin, who are

closer to the Winter season, will tan more easily and the tan will be a red-brown. But most Summers do not tan well, they burn and peel. By nature Summers are not sun worshipers. They tend to protect themselves from the sun. There are a few Summers who may appear sallow or gray, which could be due to poor health.

Summer Skin Is:
Fair with delicate pink tone
Light to medium rose beige
Deep rose beige

SUMMER EYES — Summer eyes can range from clear blue or green to gray-blue, gray-green, aquamarine, hazel or brown. Blue is the most usual eye color for a Summer. Those brown eyes we do see are a soft brown. The Summer blue eye can be a very clear blue, almost like a marble; others are a deep blue-gray with a violet tint around the pupil and a gray ring around the iris, much like the Winter eye. Green eyes found in Summer can be clear green to a gray-green with soft white or yellow radiating out from the pupil.

Hazel eyes of a Summer are a blue-green with brown and/or yellow flecks. These eyes have a chameleon-like quality of changing color depending on mood or on what color is worn.

Summer Eyes Are:
Clear blue or gray-blue
Clear green or gray-green
Aquamarine
Hazel
Soft, cool brown

SUMMER HAIR — Some Summers have very light ash blonde hair which often darkens with age. This type is a true blonde and looks good when she keeps her hair ash blonde even into late maturity. This woman can frost her hair most successfully. Many Summers were towheads as children. The light to dark brown hair of this season appears to be a "mousy" color because of the grayish cast. This hair may appear dull and lifeless when the wrong makeup is used and the wrong colors are worn, but beautiful when enhanced by wearing the right colors.

Summers gray gracefully, turning a silver gray. Summer is the only season which can frost her hair successfully, and even then only the ash blonde to medium brown should frost. Avoid over-frosting. Dark brown hair should never frost. Summers whose skin coloring is high (pink) have a lot of red pigment which will bring out red highlights in the hair when exposed to sunlight. It is very important to use an ash brown color when dying the hair to avoid the red. Summers are not redheads!

Summer Hair Is:
Light ash blonde
Medium ash blonde
Light to medium ash brown
Dark ash brown
Gray (silver)

YOUR INNER SEASON — Our observations about the Summer woman note that she is most often classic, controlled and ladylike with a soft, gentle look. She should never attempt a dramatic effect. Summers are gracious, poised and even-tempered with soft, calm voices. The Summer woman gets more done with less effort. Often artistic, she is skilled in many endeavors. She is a good listener, sincerely interested in other people. No service is too difficult for Summer to perform if she is devoted to the cause. Because she has a soft shoulder and sympathetic ear, she often gets involved in everyone's problems and caught up in the neighborhood gossip.

The Summer woman loves dainty, pretty things. She loves her home and is happy in the roles of wife, mother and homemaker. A Summer is organized, analytical, the kind of woman who would like to remake the world and everyone in it. She usually excels in domestic arts and makes a great executive secretary or office manager because she is a super organizer. She becomes involved in school, community and social organizations, and is often found as president of the PTA and other service clubs. Summers are morning people — they rise early to get a good start. The Summer woman is quite set in her ways, stubborn and hard to convince, but once converted, she remains devoted. She is pleasant and sincere, a good sport, loyal friend, devoted sweetheart and wife. She has a heart of gold.

The Summer woman is usually a fashion conservative. She has a comfort zone and is not eager to step out of it. Slow to consider a new fashion, she is usually the last to adopt it and by the time she does, it is almost out of style. Her children always get new shoes; if there is any money left in the budget, she might get around to buying herself a pair. She is a bit of a penny-pincher who thrills at news of a sale and will use a tank of gas to get there.

The Spring Woman

Springs are the golden girls. They have a yellow undertone in their skin. Many of them are descendants of the Scandinavian races, or people of the Netherlands, British Isles, Iceland and Northern Europe. Springs take great interest in the course at the Fashion Academy because they are very interested in personal appearance, theirs and everybody else's. They are delightful and enthusiastic women to have around. We always get a lift out of Springs. They are so eager to learn that they want the whole course in the first lesson.

SPRING SKIN — Ivory with gold-tone is typical of the Spring season. Some are so fair that they appear milky white, even sickly, with skin and hair the same color. Pink or peach skin has a glow to it with rosy cheeks. Springs may flush easily and have almost a redheaded ruddiness. Some Springs will freckle. A deep-peach-skinned Spring tans very easily and, if an outdoor person, will hold it all year. Light to medium beige skin has more yellow in it and looks sallow. This coloring is closest to Autumn and needs makeup to look look healthy.

Spring Skin Tones:
Pale ivory
Golden ivory
Pink or peach
Deep peach
Light to medium beige
Rosy glow

SPRING EYES — All colors of eyes are found in Spring, with more blue and fewer brown. Spring eyes range from light to dark blue. Some Springs have blue-gray eyes. These eyes may have a gray ring around the iris and a mixture of gold and white flecks around the pupil resembling granite. Many Springs have aqua (green-blue) eyes with gold flecks. Topaz, a golden yellow, is a beautiful, unusual eye color found in Spring. Golden green eyes are very common in Spring. There are few brown eyes, and those few found in Spring are light brown with gold and/or green flecks.

Spring Eyes Are:
Light to dark blue
Blue-gray
Green-blue (aqua)
Gold-green
Light gold-brown
Topaz-yellow
Hazel

SPRING HAIR — Springs are most often blonde with hair color ranging from light flaxen to a golden honey or light to medium brown with gold highlights. Spring blondes usually darken with age, but they can keep their hair blonde artificially and it looks great if not allowed to get too brassy. Some fair Springs may have had bright, carrot-red hair as babies or children. With maturity this hair will usually turn to strawberry blonde or a golden honey brown.

Some Springs with brown hair have red highlights. A few Springs are found with dark, warm brown hair.

Many Springs do not gray gracefully, but they seldom wait around to find this out. They color their hair, because the gray tones often give it a drab look. When completely gray, the hair is a soft, white-gray.

Spring Hair Is:
Flaxen blonde
Golden blonde
Strawberry blonde
Light to dark golden brown
Gray (warm)
White (warm)

YOUR INNER SEASON — Our observations of the Spring woman show her to be refreshing, exciting and fun to have around. She moves quickly and smiles easily. Friendly, animated and impulsive, Spring is casually hospitable and loves luxury. She is feminine, energetic, bubbly and unpredictable. A Spring is not usually the studious type, but never underestimate her intelligence. She may appear to be childlike and helpless, but she will be talented and capable in her own disorganized way. A Spring woman may have trouble in professional life convincing others that she means business. She needs to look feminine but never fussy, or people get the idea that she is frivolous.

Usually an extrovert, Spring is sometimes coy; she enjoys being in the limelight and can be a little self-centered.

A Spring woman has very sensitive feelings. She can be easily hurt and intimidated. Her moods fluctuate, and she may sulk when she doesn't get her way. She may seem innocent, naive, artless and dependent, but Spring knows what she is doing every minute. She is accustomed to compliments, having been pampered since babyhood. Financial security is important to her; she needs to be cared for. Spring loves children and pets and is a good-time person. Ready to go at a moment's notice, she lives for today and may lose interest in some of her projects before they are completed. She has many plans but may try to go in too many directions at one time. Daily routine bores her, a trait which may make her appear flighty. Spring is a night person — she dislikes going to bed early and loves to sleep late. Her appearance is important to her. With her delicate, natural beauty, she is ageless.

The Autumn Woman

Autumns can be a blend of any racial background of no specific origin unless you count the redheaded Irish. We often have fewer Autumns at the Academy because they are too busy to take time out for classes. Autumns always have a lot of irons in the fire.

Autumns have a yellow undertone to their skin. Most redheads are Autumns unless they have blue eyes, and then they are probably Springs. Many Autumns appear to be sallow. Unless they wear makeup they may not look good, even in their own colors. Without makeup they look like someone erased their faces. This is due to their light brows and lashes and a lack of natural color in their lips and cheeks. Most Autumns look best

with a little tan on their faces to add color. When an Autumn is sick she looks sick, almost green. Many women (especially Winters) think they are Autumns because they like, and have worn camel and beige. But in order to be an Autumn you must be able to wear all the dusty greens, rusts, yellows and golds.

AUTUMN SKIN — Some Autumns have very fair ivory skin which does not tan easily. This skin has more color and may look ruddy or florid. Any of the lighter Autumn skin tones may freckle. The beige skin, light to dark, is very sallow and the yellow undertone is more noticeable. The medium to deep beige skin tans more easily. Autumns usually tan a golden color, but the deeper beige skin when tan looks dirty.

> *Autumn Skin Tones:*
> Ivory
> Light, medium or deep peach
> Light, medium or dark beige
> Florid

AUTUMN EYES — Most Autumns have brown eyes but the brown can cover a wide spectrum — golden amber with dark brown or black flecks, to reddish-brown, light to dark, with a rich rust color circling the pupil and fading out into the darker brown of the outer iris.

Many Autumn children have very dark brown eyes, almost black-looking, but with maturity their eyes may lighten. Eyes which were brown in youth often mature with green in them or look hazel.

Autumns may have avocado-green eyes with gold flecks (cat eyes) or olive-green or olive-brown eyes.

The Autumn hazel eye will be predominantly brown with a little blue-green in it.

There are very few blue eyes found in Autumn. The eyes may be turquoise, but they will be more green than blue.

Autumn's eyes are truly the windows of her soul. Her eyes are very expressive and change with her mood. When Autumns are happy or excited, their eyes sparkle and dance. The flecks of gold make them shine.

Autumn Eyes Are:
Light to dark brown, red-brown, olive-brown
Golden-green (cat eyes)
Hazel
Turquoise

AUTUMN HAIR — Most Autumn children have golden honey blonde to light brown hair which will darken with age.

Autumns may have honey blonde to golden blonde to dishwater blonde hair. The dishwater blonde is really a drab brown with golden highlights. You will often see this color hair on young women.

Autumns might have strawberry blonde or light to medium sandy-red hair. They might also be bright carrot-tops or deep auburn. Red hair is most predominant in Autumn and most Autumns look good with red highlights in the hair, even if these highlights are artificial.

Light to dark brown hair may have gold or red highlights. The dark brown hair may be a deep chestnut with auburn highlights. Autumns do not gray gracefully. The transition period of graying is not attractive until they are completely gray because the gray mixed with their warm highlights has a dull, drab look. Their gray hair is a warm gray. Autumns don't have very much color, so when their hair fades, their skin and eyes fade also and they appear all one color. This is why makeup is important for Autumns.

An Autumn should never frost her hair. It may be highlighted by "luminizing"™ or painting, but the highlights should be subtle. Autumns usually look best if their hair is dyed a solid color with red or gold highlights. It should *never* be dyed an ash brown, for it will turn drab with a greenish cast.

Autumn Hair Is:
Honey blonde
Strawberry blonde
Bright red to deep auburn
Light to dark brown with gold
or red highlights
Deep chestnut-brown
Gray (warm)
White (warm)

YOUR INNER SEASON — After observing many Autumns over the years, the one thing that we can say about them is that it is impossible to generalize about Autumns. They are highly individual. The Autumn woman is usually extroverted but at times is quiet and reserved. Open and enthusiastic, she is trusting to the point of being gullible. She has a mercurial disposition, subject to extremes of mood. An Autumn is independent and makes a good leader. Well organized in her own haphazard way, she is a perfectionist, and no one can figure out how to do anything to suit her. She is loyal, affectionate and incurably optimistic. Sensitive to the vibes around her, she is also temperamental, mischievous and proud. The Autumn woman can be very patient if not pushed too far, but sometimes "too far" is the brink of disaster. She moves quickly and smiles easily. Friendly and impulsive, Autumn thrives on luxury. She has lots of friends but is a private person who needs time for herself. She is fun-loving with a great sense of humor. Home and family are important to her, but she likes to do her own thing and often gets bored with the daily routine. Autumn is a good career woman, creative but sometimes lacking direction. Dedicated to her current cause, she always has several projects going and bites off more than she can chew. The only trait all Autumns have in common is a trace of delightful zaniness.

Whatever season you are, you will enhance your beauty by wearing those colors that are best for you.

Those of you who may have difficulty in determining your season might benefit from the assistance of a Certified Fashion Academy color consultant.

Once your season has been determined, however, it is time to turn your attention to your body and the clothes which adorn it.

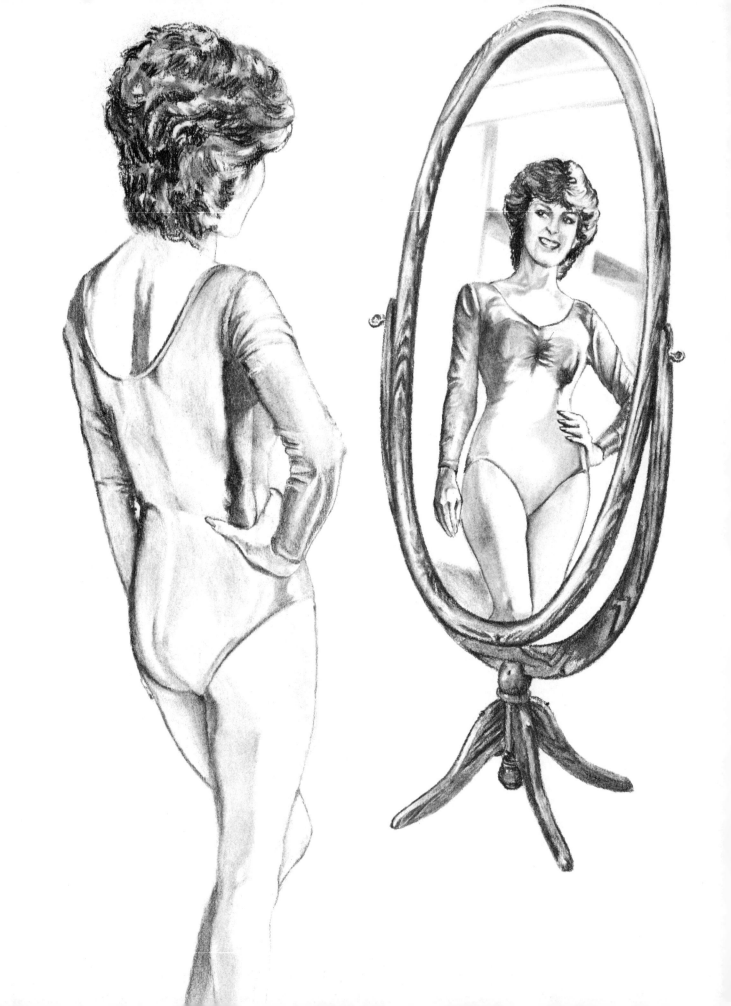

CHAPTER TWO

Body Line

YOUR FIGURE ANALYSIS

In order to choose clothing which is becoming, which makes you look and feel your best, you need to understand exactly what kind of body you are working with. It has been our experience in working with women that they rarely appreciate their good qualities and tend to dwell on their few figure problems.

American women are so intimidated by the mythical "fashion figure" that it never occurs to them that many clothing problems are attributable to short-sighted clothing manufacturers rather than to any grave deficiencies in their individual bodies.

Before you can solve a problem you must identify it. In this chapter we hope to guide you to better self-evaluation and then lead you to suggestions which will enable you to make the most of yourself.

We have found that if you accentuate your positive qualities your problems will take care of themselves.

Balance And Proportion Of The Body

If you were perfectly proportioned you could wear any style you wanted. Few people are perfectly proportioned, however. We use clothing to create the illusion of a well proportioned, balanced body. We can make the eye see anything we want it to see with clever use of line and design.

A good figure is a matter of visual proportion and balance rather than a relationship of height to weight. A good figure has a rhythmic gradation of restrained curves. The curves of a large bust, hip or thigh are abrupt changes in size, and so is a very small waist. Unrestrained curves present fitting problems and require skill in choice of design to camouflage or to create better proportion. (Ready-to-wear clothing is designed for the tall, slender, well proportioned figure with a balanced, tapered shoulder, a small bust and a tapered hip.) A good figure has good posture and properly fitted foundation garments. A good figure has a balanced hair style in keeping with the body as a whole.

THE REAL YOU — Stand in front of a full-length mirror, clothed only in bra and underpants. Be objective and honest. Your aim is to make a visual evaluation of your body proportion and balance as determined by your bone structure, the distribution of your flesh, your muscle structure and your adipose or fatty tissue. Use a hand-held mirror to observe your posture and body structure from the side and rear. If you have long hair, put it up off the neck for a more accurate evaluation. Posture is a vital factor and will often determine how good you will look in your clothes.

To develop good posture, practice standing correctly — lift the diaphragm, keeping the wrinkles out of your midriff. Lifting the diaphragm puts the shoulders in proper position. Without

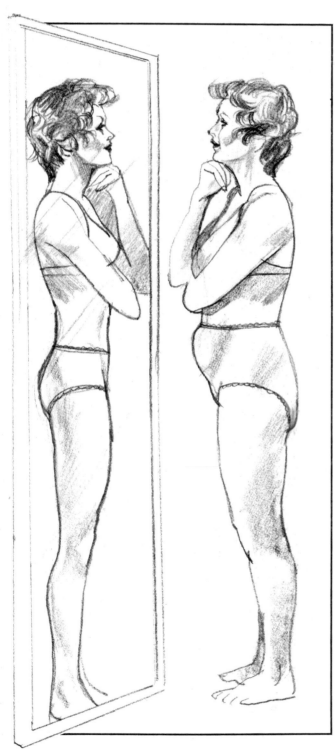

Mirror Myopia

even thinking about your shoulders, they will fall into alignment, back and down. Rotate your hips forward — you can get a feel for this by tightening the buttock muscles as if you were holding a quarter between your buttocks. Keep your knees flexed, not locked, when standing. Flexed knees are more attractive and allow a more relaxed, less tiring standing position. Keep your eyes directed at eye level. If the eyes fall, everything goes. Walk by swinging the legs from the hip, not the knees, and you will glide as you walk.

It is very difficult to be objective about oneself. If you have trouble being objective, poke two eyeholes in a paper bag and place it over your head. Then evaluate the body you see in the mirror before you.

You may wish to record your findings.

BODY TYPE — This is a term used to describe the size of the skeletal structure. There are no particular criteria for determining an ideal. The bone structure should balance with the body as a whole, primarily in respect to height, width and adipose tissue. Determining body type by wrist circumference alone is insufficient. You need to consider the width of the shoulder, the fullness of the chest and the thickness of the shoulder from front to back.

Body Types Are:
Slender
Medium
Sturdy

Height

Apparent height has to do not only with how many inches tall you are, but also with the relationship between your height and your width. A thin woman appears taller than a sturdy woman. Generally, 5′6″ (167.6 cm) and over is considered tall; 5′4″ (162.6 cm) to 5′5″ (166.3 cm) is considered average. Anyone 5′3″ (160 cm) and under is considered short.

Women Are:
 Tall
 Average
 Short

Face Shape

The ideal face shape is an oval. We strive to create the illusion of an oval by hair styling. To determine your face shape, hold hair back with a head band, close one eye and trace your face as reflected in the bathroom mirror with a sliver of soap. Another method is to hold a long pencil near the outer corner of one eye keeping the pencil perpendicular. Observe the outline of the face which extends beyond the pencil, particularly the location of the width. With maturity, an oval face can appear square due to the relaxation of the flesh along the jaw line.

Faces Can Be:
 Oval
 Oblong or rectangular
 Round
 Square
 Triangle
 Heart or inverted triangle
 Diamond

Head Size

Traditionally, the ideal figure has been considered to be eight heads tall, which is a good proportion. This means that the total length of the head, not including hair, will divide into the total height eight times. The tall, model-type figure often conforms to this proportion. A figure with a small head appears to be taller and thinner than one with a large head. The figure in the fashion ad is as much as twelve heads tall and far too thin. Students at the Fashion Academy average about seven and one-half heads tall, which is a good proportion. The impact of this proportion concerns the head, specifically the hair style, and

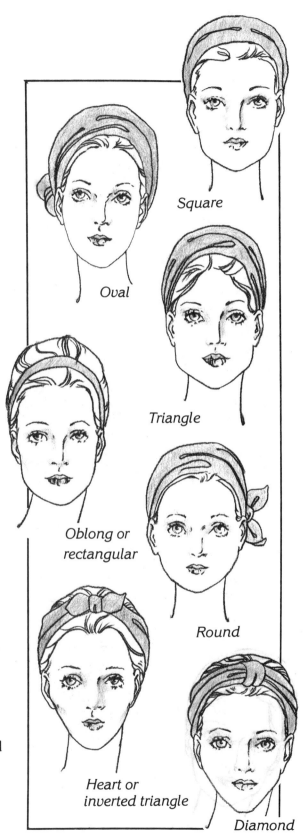

Oval

Square

Triangle

Oblong or rectangular

Round

Heart or inverted triangle

Diamond

helps determine whether the hair should be styled in a fuller or more compact style.

The apparent size of your head is visual. Delicate or prominent facial features will also influence how large your head appears. Evaluate your head size according to your own observations or feelings about yourself.

Heads May Be:
Small
Proportioned
Large

Head Position

Ideally, when viewed from the side, if we dropped a string through the middle of the head, it would fall just behind the lobe of the ear, bisect the shoulder and fall down the middle of a perfectly aligned body. Most people carry their head forward. This is a congenital condition which is aggravated by poor posture, lack of muscle tone in the upper back and possibly your occupation. If your head is set forward, you must be especially conscious of your posture and utilize collars, scarves and neck styling to create the illusion of a well aligned head.

A fleshy deposit on the prominent vertebrae at the base of the neck could indicate the possible future development of a "dowager's hump." This condition is familial. There are indications that good posture, proper exercise, good diet and attention to the hormone balance, especially in mature women, can preclude development of this unfortunate condition.

Head Positions Are:
Aligned
Forward

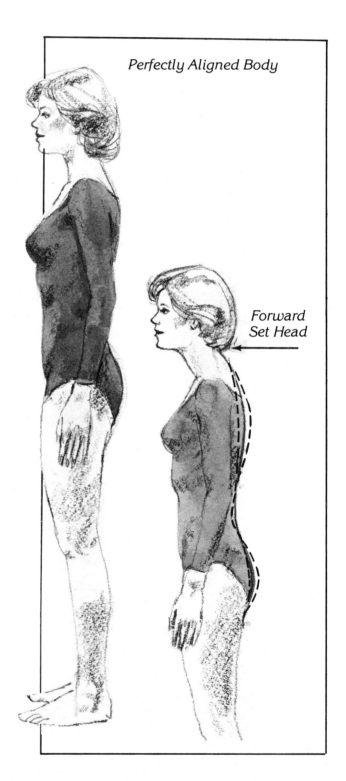

Perfectly Aligned Body

Forward Set Head

Upper And Lower Back

The ideal upper back should be slightly rounded. Posture, bone structure and adipose tissue can contribute to a too-rounded upper back. Thinness or an angular bone structure can make the upper back appear flat.

The term "lower back" refers to the back of the midriff, waist and upper hip. We describe many women as "swayback," which means that they have a concave area above a shapely derriere. Others, particularly if they have flat bottoms, will be quite flat in the lower back. Neither could be particularly described as the "ideal." A moderate curve looks better in pants, moderately flat looks better in a dress. The condition is of interest primarily in respect to fitting alterations, which may be needed for either type (see Chapter 4, page 77).

Upper Backs Are:
  Flat
  Slightly round
  Round

Lower Backs Are:
  Flat
  Slightly round
  Round
  Swayback

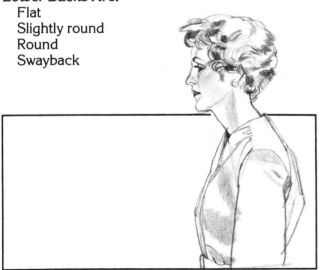

Neck Length

The ideal neck length is visual, having to do not only with its actual length but with its sturdiness or slimness as well. The position of the head affects apparent neck length. A forward-set head has a shortening effect on the neck. Square shoulders will make the neck appear shorter, but a very sloped shoulder will make the neck appear longer. The width and length of your neck must be considered in choosing necklines and collars.

Necks Are:
  Short
  Medium
  Long

They Are:
  Slender
  Sturdy

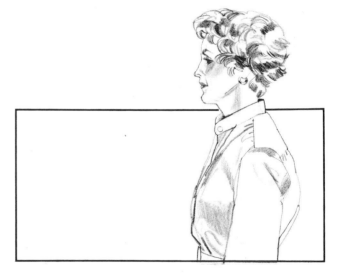

A forward set head or a Dowager's Hump can be less noticeable with the addition of a collar in back.

Shoulder Width

Ideally, the shoulders will be as wide or slightly wider than the hips. They should also balance with the size of the bust. An individual with good shoulders can gain weight without it being particularly noticeable, while the one with narrow shoulders will show every extra pound. In evaluating the width of your shoulders you must remember that your shoulders will look different when you are wearing pants than they will when you are wearing a skirt because hips look wider in pants. When the hips look wider, the shoulders look narrower.

Your shoulders may appear to be of ideal size from the waist up, but if you have large hips, you must consider yourself as having narrow shoulders.

A full bust may be balanced with broad shoulders, but the same size bust would appear to be much larger with narrow shoulders. A person who has broad shoulders and slim hips appears to be taller than she is because she is carrying the width of her body higher. The closer your width is to the ground, as with broad hips, the shorter you look.

Shoulder Width:
Balanced
Broad
Narrow
Full busted

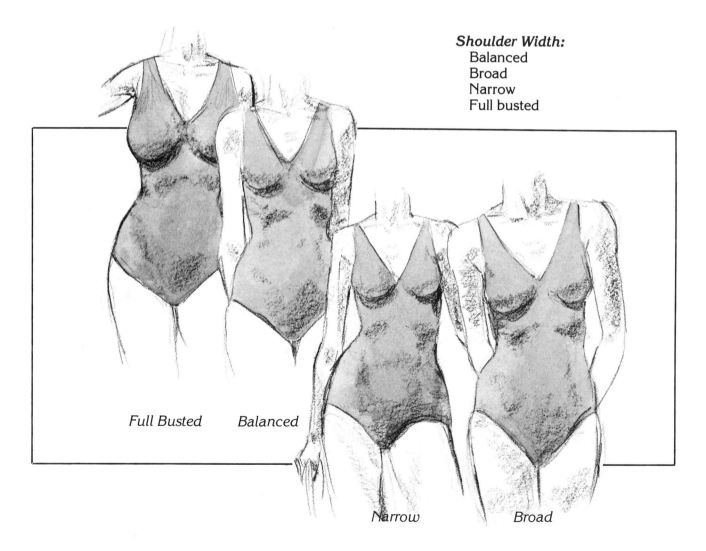

Full Busted   Balanced

Narrow   Broad

Shoulder Slope

All ready-to-wear garments and all patterns assume that there is a two-inch drop from the base of the neck to the tip of the shoulders. We find that most people's shoulders do not drop that much. They are more square. If your shoulders vary sufficiently from the hypothetical "norm" either in being too square or too sloped, you will have a fitting problem and need to consider shoulder slope in style selection. If your shoulders conform approximately to a two-inch drop, we call them tapered. More than a two-inch drop we call sloped. If your shoulders are more square, estimate the different degree of squareness.

Bust Size

The apparent size of the bust can be deceiving. The shape and size of the chest under the breast affects its apparent size. A "pigeon" chest or a full bone structure in the chest area can make a small breast appear larger. Generally speaking, an A cup bra size would be small; a B or C cup, medium; and a D or above would be large.

A very large bust is almost always out of proportion with the rest of the body, resulting in nearly insoluble fitting problems. A large breast often causes backache, deep grooves in the

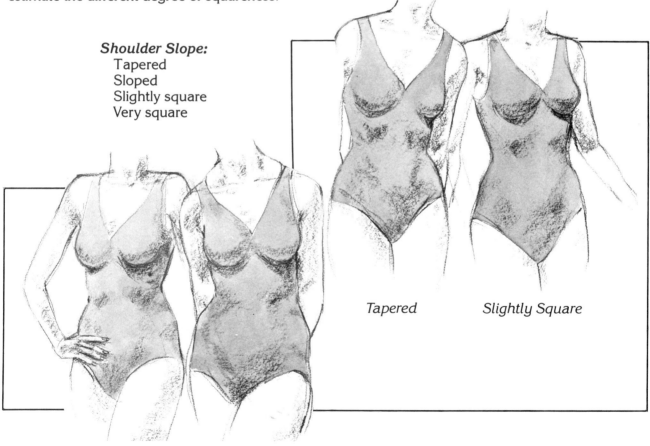

Shoulder Slope:
Tapered
Sloped
Slightly square
Very square

Tapered   *Slightly Square*

Very Square   *Sloped*

shoulder due to the weight on the bra strap, and poor posture. Large breasts are particularly susceptible to health problems. The woman with a very large bust might consider mammoplasty or breast reduction. Mammoplasty is no longer considered cosmetic surgery. Most good health insurance policies cover it. Mammoplasty, if needed, will take ten years off your apparent age, improve posture and health, to say nothing about providing comfort and greater ease in obtaining properly fitted clothing.

Bust Sizes Are:
  Small
  Medium
  Large

Bust Location

On the youthful figure, the crown (fullest point) of the bust is about 1 to 1½ (4-5 cm) below the underarm. As one matures, or the bust grows larger, it tends to drop. A high line gives a youthful look. One indication of a matronly figure is a droopy bustline. A low bust also shortens the midriff. A figure with a thick waist will look thicker if the bust is low. Raising the bustline to its proper position will add length to the midriff, making the body appear slimmer. The position of the crown of the bust is also very important. The main objection to the "natural" or sweater bra is that it allows the breasts to swing out to the sides and drop, which broadens the torso and does nothing to enhance the contour of the breast. A firm, rounded bustline is pleasing. A droopy, sagging bustline is not. Mature bodies need well-fitted bras of good construction. A woman who goes braless for any reason is encouraging tissue breakdown and will someday have to pay the price.

When purchasing bras, choose a well stocked store with trained saleswomen who know their merchandise and understand your needs. The cost of a bra is the same whether you buy it off a counter without even trying it on or have the service of a trained clerk. Tell her you have come for a fitting and explain what you hope to achieve with your new bra.

Take with you, to the store, a blouse which buttons down the front. Before trying a new garment, place a safety pin on the crown of the bust on the blouse while wearing your old bra. After you have put on the new one, put the blouse back on and check what the new garment is doing to the contour of your breasts by comparing the location of the crown of your bust with the safety pins. Any bra is only as good as the fitter.

Bust Location Is:
  Good
  Low

Midriff

The more slender the midriff is, the longer it will appear. The rib cage determines the size of the midriff and whether it looks wide from side to side or from front to back. The bust location also affects the apparent length of the midriff.

Midriffs Are:
  Slender
  Full
  Long
  Medium
  Short

Waistline

To determine the location of your waistline, fasten a one-inch-wide belt snugly around your waist. The bottom of the belt is your correct waistline location.

Tiny waistlines are gone forever. Women will never again subject themselves to the physical restraint which was largely responsible for the eighteen-inch waistlines of our ancestors. Physical freedom of the female body has pretty much kept pace with women's political freedom. Women today are politically liberated, and freedom from the restraint of clothing has gone about as far as it can go. In contrast to Scarlett O'Hara's sixteen-inch (41 cm) waistline, a twenty-five-inch (64 cm) waistline today is very small. Twenty-seven (69 cm) to twenty-eight inches (71 cm) is about average. The size of the waistline is influenced by the location of the hip bone, the location and size of the rib cage, the amount of adipose tissue and the type of undergarments worn. The absence of restrictive undergarments has allowed the body to develop according to nature's intent. The ideal waist is long and moderately slim, forming a slender connection between midriff and hip.

A slender rib cage with a lower hip bone (tapered hip) results in a small waist. Even with heavy thighs this figure retains the long, slim-waisted look. A wider, lower rib cage in combination with a high hip bones results in a thick waist. Because of the placement of the bone structure, all the dieting in the world will not produce a small waistline. In addition, any weight gain in this high-hipped figure will deposit itself on the hip bones, further thickening the appearance of the waistline.

Apparent waist length is visual and has to do with total body proportion. A short or long waist becomes a problem, however when you do not conform to ready-to-wear waist lengths. Choice of proper silhouette (see Chapter 3) can balance poor proportion. Two piece garments will solve the fit problem.

Panty hose are a culprit in distorting the waistline. (Tight elastic produces twin rolls, above and below.) If the hose are too short, the elastic rides across the flesh of the upper hip, pushing the roll of fat up. It is imperative to search until you discover a design or brand of hose in the correct length for your legs.

A small waistline at one time was considered to be the epitome of feminity. It is no longer a criterion for a good figure. The measurement is not important, appearance is.

Hips

For purposes of clarity in this discussion, let us first establish some "body language." We will identify the upper part of the hip area as "hip" and the lower part as "thigh."

Nature has produced two distinctive types of hip bone structure in the female. The first has a high hip bone set close to the waistline with the structure of the lower pelvic bone more flat, resulting in a flat thigh. We will call this type a *high hip* and a *flat thigh.*

The second type finds the hip bone farther from the waistline and the pelvic structure more protrusive in the thigh area. We will label this type a *tapered hip* and a *full thigh.*

IDENTIFYING YOUR HIP STRUCTURE — When we talk about the hip bone, we are referring to the corner of the pelvic bone which you can feel on the front of your body. It is a rounded bone and lies five to eight inches from the center front. It may be parallel with the navel or it can be much lower. The high hip bone is often more prominent and easier to feel than the tapered hip bone.

If you are unable to identify your hip bone type, run your hand down the side of your hip and feel your thigh. The high hip bone is usually accompanied by a flat thigh while the tapered hip bone nearly always has a prominent thigh bone. It is possible, through addition of adipose tissue, to have both a high hip *and* a full thigh.

HIGH HIP — The high hip falls closer to the waistline. This bone structure typically has a flat thigh. Any excess weight on this figure will deposit on the high hip bone front and back and on the tummy just below the waist in front. The "spare tire" look comes with maturity. The high hip body type frequently finds that the rib cage is closer to the waist and the waistline, consequently, is thick. This type rarely has a small waist. The legs appear longer because of the flat thigh. With maturity there may be a drop of flesh on the side back, giving the illusion of a full thigh, but this is flesh, not bone, and does not change the hip type. It just compounds your problem when it comes to finding flattering styles.

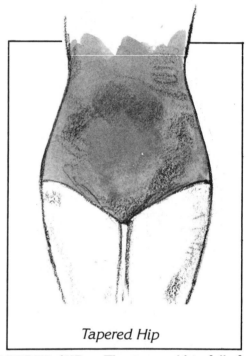

Tapered Hip

TAPERED HIP — The tapered hip falls farther from the waistline and typically has the full thigh caused by protruding bone structure low on the side. This figure type puts any excess weight directly on the thigh bone but retains the tapered hip, as we call it, unless weight gain is extreme. This type more typically has the rib cage farther above the waist, resulting in a longer, slimmer midriff, slimmer waist and lower tummy. The legs will seem shorter because of the fuller thigh and the longer-appearing torso. With maturity the bottom will drop, further accentuating the full thigh.

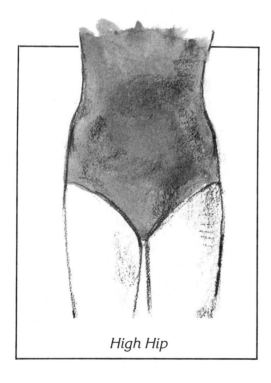

High Hip

IN-BETWEEN HIP — Some women have a hip which is balanced between the two extremes. An example would be a slender midriff with a high round hip, or a tapered hip which has a slim thigh. These fortunate individuals have no problem in this area in clothing selection. On the other hand, those who carry more adipose tissue would have fatty pads on a tapered hip bone or fat saddles on a flat thigh bone. Nowhere on the body is weight of more consequence than in the hip area.

Hips Are:
High
Tapered
In-between

Hip Line

One other area of the body which is very important for you to identify is the hip line or the break of the leg. This is where your body bends when you lift your knee, where the leg bone fits into the hip socket. When a woman is young, the hip line is the fullest part of the hip. As you mature, however, the flesh drops, often causing the fullest part to be lower on the body. For purposes of determining lengths of tops and jackets, however, we will determine your hip line by where your body bends or breaks when you lift your knee.

Tummy

On the high hip body type, any weight gain will settle first on the high hip bones. This also holds true for the location of the tummy. The high hip body type will have a high round tummy, just below the waistline. This figure type has a tendency to develop a tummy if there is any excess weight at all or with maturity.

The appearance of a full tummy is often due more to the hollow of the waistline directly above the abdomen rather than the tummy itself. If you fill in the waistline hollow with a tie belt, or in the case of slacks, with a center front zipper, the effect is of a flatter stomach. This type of waistline-tummy combination demands a looser waistband so that the waistband does not cup in above the stomach, making it appear larger.

Some bodies develp a barrel shape (full in front midriff, waist and tummy area.) On the tapered hip body type, the round tummy, if there is one, will be lower on the body.

Tummies Are:
Flat
Round
Barrel-shaped

Bottoms

As the bottom loses its muscle tone, it will drop. The downward pull of gravity starts taking effect shortly after age twenty-five. The dropping flesh gives a squared-off bottom look, much the

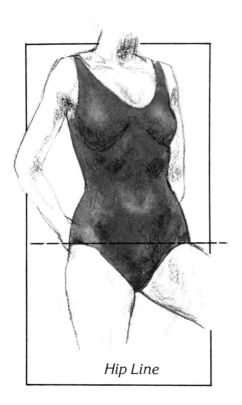

Hip Line

same as we see in faces as the jaw loses its tone. Exercise and keeping slim will help, but age inevitably will take its toll. The moment of truth comes when you find that all your bathing suits creep up in back. No, the bathing suits have not shrunk, nor have you grown — your bottom has just dropped. When the bottom drops, it causes a hollow area on the side back of the leg just above where the thigh bone is connected to the hip socket. A dropped bottom will also have a shortening effect on the legs. On the tapered hip person, any weight gain in the thigh area will add to the "saddlebag" look.

A word about undergarments: When choosing panties, a cotton crotch is best for health. Never wear bikini panties under slacks or knit dresses to avoid the dreadful roll they produce. In buying pantyhose, fit is critical in length and in the waist elastic. Try different brands until you find the one cut for your dimensions. The sizing of different brands is not uniform. If the elastic is too tight, clip it halfway through in several places to loosen it. Panty hose are not good under slacks. Wear knee-high hose or pant liners. Time was when "ladies wore girdles." That has changed with the advent of panty hose, but all ladies still need a girdle under clingy knits to control quivering flesh. Choose a long-line or all-in-one if you wish to trim your thighs or tend to develop rolls from a skimpier style. Modern girdles are of light construction and cannot take the place of a diet. Worn too tight they cause more problems than they solve. This is another situation where a trained salesperson will help you avoid purchasing the wrong type of garment.

Bottoms run the gamut from round as a bowling ball, to delightfully medium, to flat as a boy's. Medium round looks better in pants, while medium flat looks better in skirts.

Bottoms Are:
High
Dropped
Round
Medium
Flat

Legs

The length of the legs is visual and has to do with total body proportion. Many women who are short automatically assume they have short legs, and tall people decide theirs are long. This is not necessarily true. Experience in measuring thousands of women has proven that shortness or tallness is due to the fact that many women's height or lack of it is found in the hip and midriff area rather than in the legs themselves. If you were to measure the length of your legs from where the body bends when you lift your knee (where the leg is connected to the hip socket), the legs will be found to be longer than the upper body.

The most important consideration is that *your leg* balances with *your body*. The shape of your hip and your adipose tissue has great visual effect on the apparent length of your leg. The leg of a high, round hip body with a flat thigh will appear much longer than the leg of a woman who has a tapered hip and a full thigh. This explains why the high hipped, flat thigh figure looks best in pants. Whatever the actual measurement may be, the proportion is purely visual.

Leg Lengths Are:
Balanced
Long
Short

Arms

If your figure is in good balance, the elbow will fit neatly into your waistline and the middle knuckle of your thumb will be even with your crotch.

The flesh of the well proportioned upper arm is fairly straight. Excess adipose tissue makes it rounded. A full upper arm is almost impossible to camouflage in anything but a loose-fitting sleeve. A small wrist and a slender forearm give the appearance of being longer. Small wrists will also make the hands appear larger.

Few women are shaped like fashion models, many of whom are 5′8″ and weigh 100 pounds. Fashion models have figure problems, but they have learned to camouflage them. Being tall and thin might make clothing choice easier, but you can also look good in your clothes if you accurately evaluate your body and then learn to select the proper garments to make the most of your good points.

Length Of Arms Are:
Short
Balanced
Long

Upper Arms Are:
Full
Slender

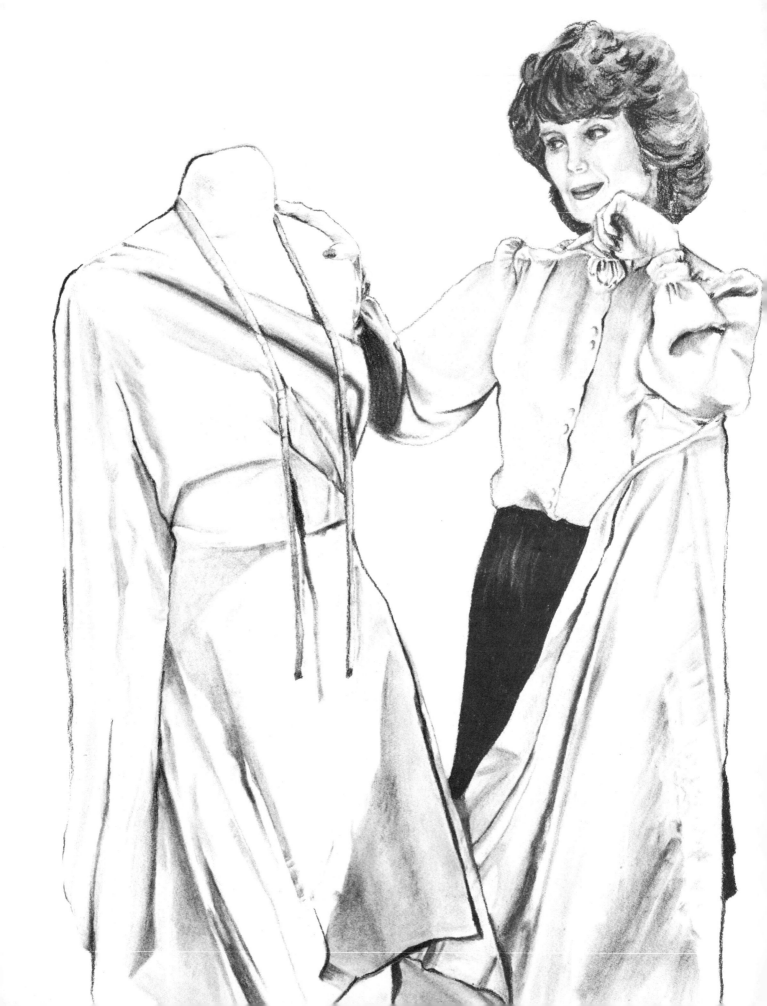

CHAPTER THREE

Clothes Line

CHOOSING YOUR BEST STYLE

fter completing your self-appraisal in Chapter 2, you now know exactly the shape the real you is in. Our next endeavor is to find the right line in the clothes you purchase or make which will accentuate your positives and hide your negatives.

There are two basic components to any garment design: structural and applied. Structural design refers to the basic shape of the garment as determined by the "shape controllers." Shape controllers include seams, darts, flares, tucks, gathers, etc. — anything which contributes to the shape of the garment or the way in which it hangs on the body. Applied design is added to make the garment more interesting, add style, or to help create the illusion of a well-proportioned body.

We have taken all contemporary clothing and divided it into five basic silhouettes or structural designs. They all start with either a shift or a princess — a garment either has seams or it doesn't. If we then place a horizontal seam above the waist, at the waist, or below the waist, we create the other three silhouettes. Your body proportion determines which of these silhouettes will be most becoming.

Structural Design - Five Basic Silhouettes

I. SHIFT

The true shift has shoulder seams and side seams. It is designed to hang from the shoulder.

The shift looks best on the figure with narrow hips or one whose shoulders balance the hips and bust. The shift may be straight, shaped or A-line. The tent, float, muu-muu, caftan, etc., are variations of this silhouette.

STRAIGHT SHIFT — The straight shift hangs from the underarm to the hem. When it is slim, it emphasizes narrow hips and camouflages a thick waist. Whether or not you belt your shift should be determined by the size and location of your waistline. Generally, the high-hipped, flat high figure will not belt the shift, preferring to emphasize her slim hips. The tapered hip figure will belt her shift to show her slim waist. Women with spare-tire middles or very short waists can often create the illusion of better balance by belting the shift and making the bodice blouse a little. This seems to camouflage the waistline. The belted shift looks best in a soft, drapey fabric, worn loose. The tapered hip with a moderate thigh can wear the straight shift if it is very loose and belted.

SHAPED SHIFT — A shaped shift is fitted in the side seams under the arms and through the midriff, and then it flares at the hem. The best ones have a center front and back seam which is also flared. The shaped shift needs to be belted. The broad-hipped, narrow-shouldered woman must use caution with this silhouette unless her outfit has some design detail which will broaden her shoulders to balance her hips.

61

TENT, FLOAT, CAFTAN SHIFT, ETC. — The full-cut shift hangs from the shoulder or bustline. This type of shift is best worn in a soft, drapey fabric, reaching to the floor. Street length in this version is attractive in very soft, thin fabric. It can hide a multitude of sins. The style is great for the mother-to-be or the very heavy woman.

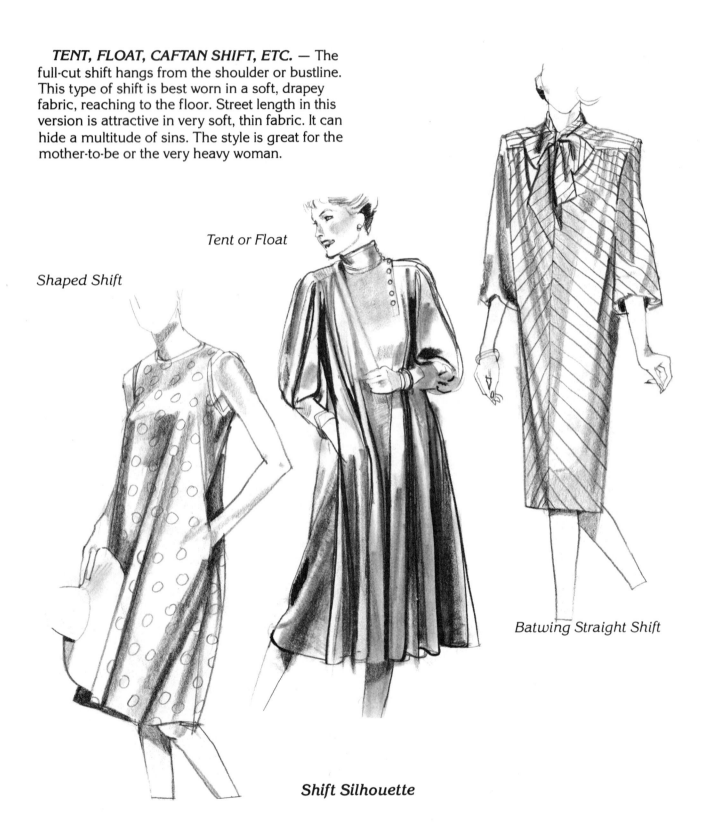

Tent or Float

Shaped Shift

Batwing Straight Shift

Shift Silhouette

Princess Silhouette

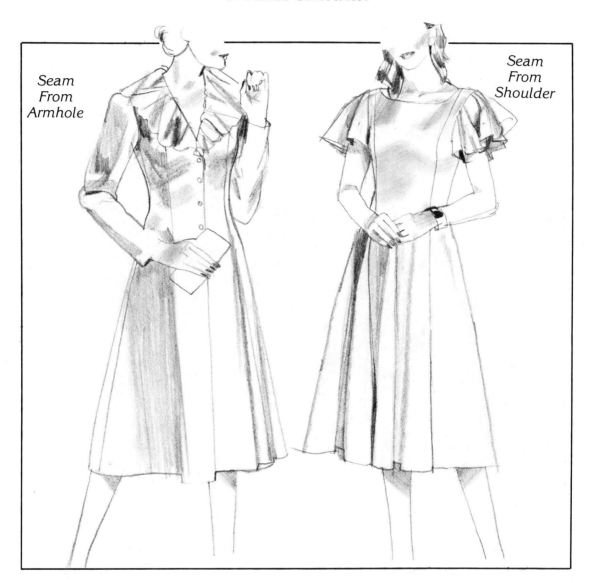

Seam
From
Armhole

Seam
From
Shoulder

II. PRINCESS

The Princess silhouette is becoming on all body types. The princess has shaped seaming. The seam can originate at the shoulder or at the arm's eye (armhole). This silhouette can also be achieved with a series of darts or tucks. For the most slimming effect, the center panel should be no wider than the space between the crowns of the bust, unless broken by a center seam or placket. The princess is more slimming if it is not too tight and when the accent of fit is in the midriff rather than the waistline. The amount of fullness in the skirt should be determined by your body proportion and personality. If you are short it cannot be too full; if you are animated, you need room to move fast. If the princess is too narrow in the skirt you can look matronly.

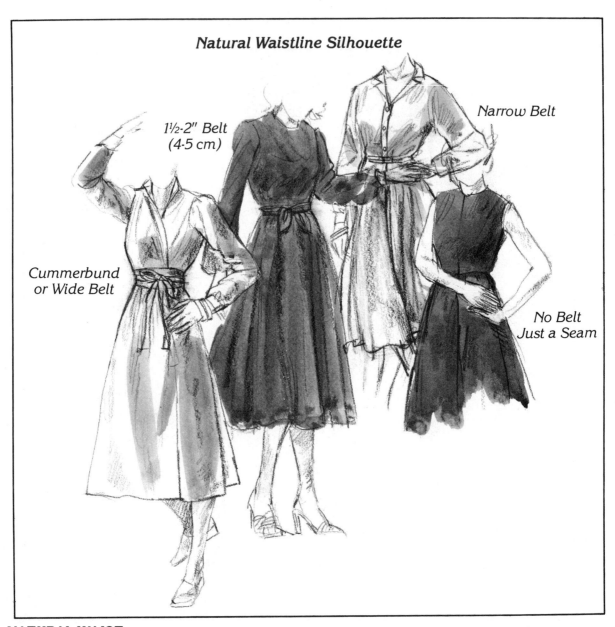

Natural Waistline Silhouette

Cummerbund or Wide Belt

1½-2" Belt (4-5 cm)

Narrow Belt

No Belt Just a Seam

III. NATURAL WAIST

Almost everyone can wear a natural waistline depending on the style. It is super on the slim-waisted, narrow midriff, tapered hip body. A small waist can wear a belt which is wide or thick, matching or in contrast. A thicker waist can create the illusion of a small waist by using a wider belt, about 1½-2 inches (4-5 cm), in self or matching fabric, and with soft fullness in the skirt. The styling in the skirt depends on the hip.

A high hip needs darts or soft gathers. If the waist is long, the belt can be raised for a slimmer, more well-proportioned look. If your waist is thick or you have a high hip, wear the belt a little loose. To make your waist look smaller, your hips look slimmer and your tummy flatter, raise your belt from ½ to 1 inch (1-3 cm) above your natural waistline. It is amazing — an instant five-pound weight loss!

IV. RAISED WAIST

This silhouette is becoming on most figures. It will make a short woman look taller and slimmer, and it gives the tall woman opportunity to add trim or contrast on the skirt. The raised waist is a very youthful line. It will look best if the line drops a little in the back. Keep the line within a few inches of the waist. If the line is slanted, it has a more slimming effect. If the line is directly under the bust, it becomes an Empire, which is good only on a youthful figure with a small, high bustline. If fullness is released from under the bust, you will look pregnant. The garment should skim the body at the rib cage. A natural waist can be visually raised with a wider self belt worn above the waistline, with a midriff band, or with trim. The angle of the high waist seam can influence apparent shoulder width — up and out to widen, down to narrow. The length of the waist — long or short — can be completely camouflaged by the raised waist silhouette.

The broad-shouldered, full-busted figure should observe the following rules:

1. If the seam is straight and the sleeve is short, the neckline must be narrowed and deepened.

2. If the neck is high and the sleeve is short, the seam must be curved down in front and dropped in back.

3. If the neck is high and the seam is straight, the sleeve must be long or the **garment** must be sleeveless.

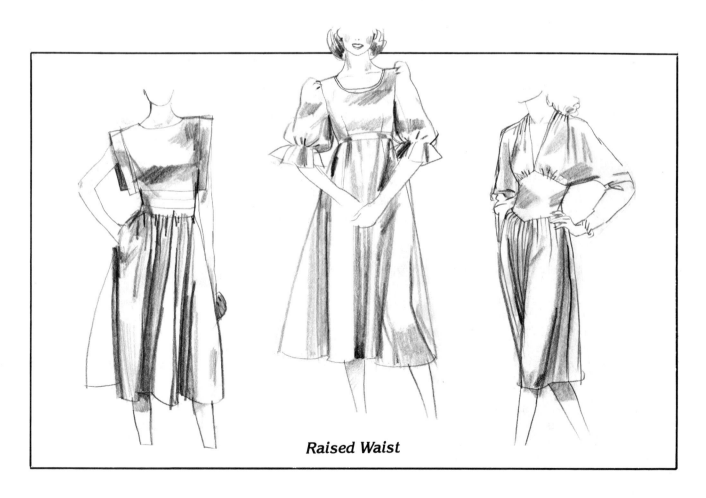

Raised Waist

65

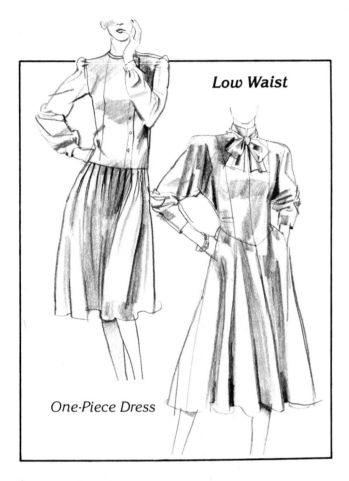

Low Waist

One-Piece Dress

small, chubby woman and is enjoyed by the thin or well proportioned figure as well. The two-piece dress is the only style that some women who have a very full midriff and tummy (barrel shape) can wear.

The overblouse should come to the hip bone or the hip line depending on your height. Any lower than the hip line looks matronly. The tops of two-piece dresses in ready-to-wear are invariably too long and must be shortened for proper proportion. The skirt should have some movement achieved with A-line, gores, pleats or flare. The top can be belted or not, following the same general rules as with the shift silhouette.

The two-piece dress looks best when done in a soft fabric with the top and skirt matching.

V. LOW WAIST

ONE-PIECE DRESS — *This silhouette is the hardest of all to wear unless you are medium to tall, well proportioned, with a tapered hip, slender midriff and a flat tummy.* The location of the line is determined by where the fullness of the hip is found. On most figures the line should fall between the hip bone and the hip line. If you have any tummy at all, the one-piece low waist dress is a dangerous choice of silhouettes. The very low seam as in the Twenties flapper look takes a tall, slender, sophisticated woman to carry it off.

TWO-PIECE DRESS — *Surprisingly, the two-piece version of the low-waist dress is one of the easiest silhouettes to wear. It looks good on the very tall, large woman. It is becoming on the*

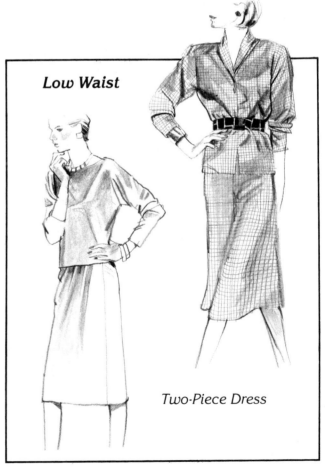

Low Waist

Two-Piece Dress

Structural Design - Silhouettes For Jackets

The two primary considerations in choice of a jacket are *shape* and *length*. The length of the jacket is determined by body proportion. Most women can wear a jacket which falls somewhere between the hip bone and the hip line with a skirt. A crotch-length jacket looks better with pants on most women. Taller women (5'6" [167.6 cm] or over) have sufficient height to wear a crotch-length jacket with a skirt. Fingertip (thigh) length jackets should be worn only by taller, slimmer girls.

SHORTER SHAPED JACKET — This suit jacket is a classic because it is the most becoming. The length should come between the hip bone and the hip line when worn with a skirt. The shorter woman must wear this jacket for proper proportion with a skirt. This is not the best jacket to wear with pants. To look good with a shorter jacket, pants should be of a looser cut in the hip and tummy and should be worn by a slender girl.

LONGER SHAPED (BLAZER) JACKET —The jacket typically worn with pants, this classic is good on almost all figures. To wear the longer shaped jacket with pants, it should come to the crotch in front. Tall women (5'6" [167.6 cm] or over) can wear this length with skirts also. Shorter women will have better proportion with a shorter jacket worn with skirts. The large-hipped figure should have the jacket loose at the hip line to give the illusion of a smaller hip. A woman with a long, slim midriff and low, tapered hip may need waistline detail (belt, top stitching or pockets) to avoid a long "stringbean" look.

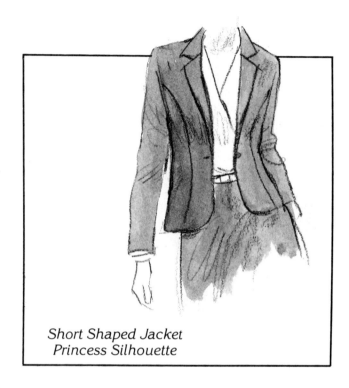

Short Shaped Jacket
Princess Silhouette

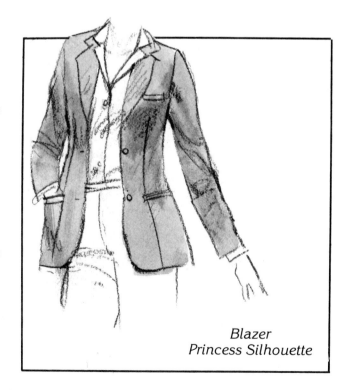

Blazer
Princess Silhouette

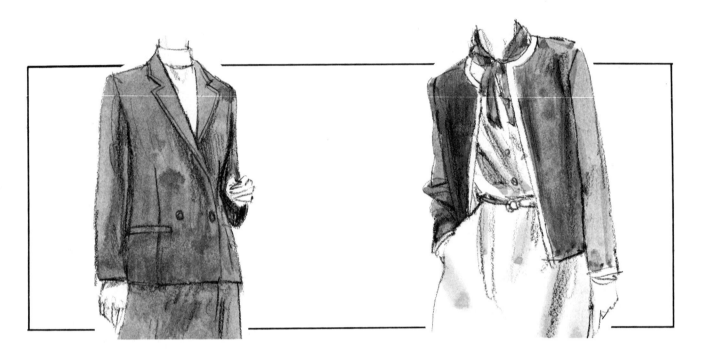

*Double-breasted Jacket
Could Be Either Princess or Shift*

*Box Jacket
Shift Silhouette*

BOX JACKET — This jacket is a straight shift, basically boxy with some shaping in the side seams. The box worn straight is best on the figure where the shoulders balance the hip and where the waist may be thick. A high-hipped, slim thigh figure can wear this jacket with a straight skirt. On the tapered hip, full thigh figure, the box jacket looks best belted and worn with an A-line skirt.

DOUBLE-BREASTED JACKET — This jacket can be a poor choice because it places six layers of fabric across the tummy and does not look good unless kept buttoned, which few women are inclined to do. The double-breasted jacket is best on the Classic or Dramatic woman with a well-proportioned body. The width between the rows of buttons can be critical. Close together, they are slimming; widely spaced, they could broaden. The double-breasted jacket could be a poor choice for your basic wardrobe because it does not combine well with other skirts and dresses. We consider it an extra in the wardrobe.

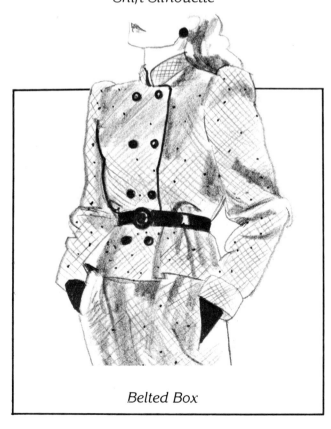

Belted Box

JACKET LENGTHS — A jacket which is curved on the bottom appears to be shorter than a jacket of the same length which is straight on the bottom. A jacket which is curved on the bottom makes the legs appear longer and is a better choice for most women, especially with pants. A jacket which is straight on the bottom should be worn a little shorter or belted. Jackets should always have ample hip room. Belting a jacket creates a peplum effect which can be very flattering to the hip.

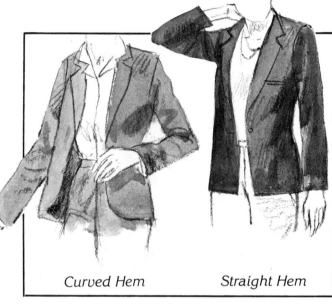

Curved Hem   *Straight Hem*

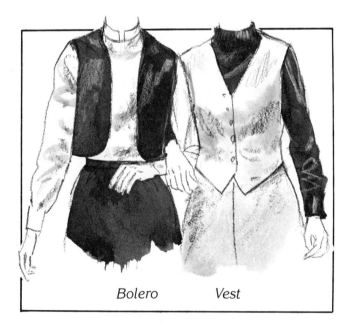

Bolero   *Vest*

VESTS AND BOLEROS — *Vests* are worn for a little added warmth or for more flare in the outfit. Care should be used to avoid looking as if you had a scrap of fabric left from your skirt which you decided to whip up into a vest. Vests should have good applied design and fit well. Vests are shaped (princess silhouette) and should reach below the waistline far enough to avoid having the blouse show underneath. The arm's eye (armhole) of your vest should come to the natural crease line where the arm joins to the shoulder. Those which are cut back in a large arm's eye make the back appear too broad and display too many seamlines when worn over a blouse. Vests combine well with any style of skirt.

Boleros add flare to a youthful costume. They are straight (shift silhouette), boxy little garments which look best if they end just above the waistline. Follow the same rule for the arm's eye as with a vest. A successful look with a bolero combines a gathered skirt topped with a wider belt or cummerbund to accentuate a slim waist. Boleros are more of a fad item than vests. They are less flattering and can be worn successfully by fewer people. Boleros are not for the full-busted figure.

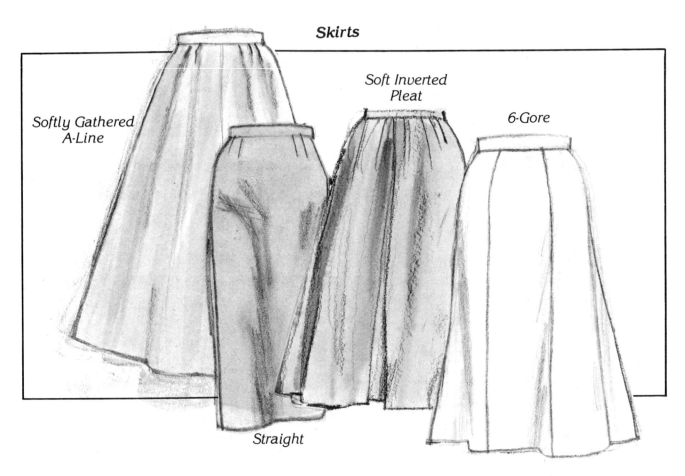

Skirts

Softly Gathered A-Line

Soft Inverted Pleat

6-Gore

Straight

Structural Design - Silhouettes For Skirts

In choosing skirt styles, follow the same basic rules as in dress silhouettes. Of most importance is the shape of your hip and waistline.

Soft fabric drapes well and is more becoming on more figure types. A skirt of soft or sheer fabric can be fuller and still be slimming. Bulky or stiff fabric adds pounds. Plaids are never slimming. Skirts cut on a true bias hug your bumps and lumps, and the zippers always bulge. If blouses are to be tucked in, skirts should have more ease. Waistbands loosely fitted will make the waist appear smaller and avoid bulges in the tummy, midriff and upper hip. A flared skirt gives the illusion of a smaller waist. Scale fullness or flare to height and weight.

As a general rule, stitched pleats should release at the hip line, kick pleats above the knee. A center-front, soft, unpressed, inverted pleat released at the waistline is very slimming. Slits can be vulgar if released too high. Always sit down to check for modesty.

STRAIGHT — This skirt is a shift silhouette, and it looks best on the figure which has a high hip and a slender thigh. Soft gathers in place of darts at the waist can be an effective camouflage for high, round hips or a round tummy. The straight skirt combines well with the box jacket. If you have a full thigh or derriere, the straight skirt must be very loose for camouflage. Center front and back seams are slimming. Personality can dictate styling such as kick pleats or slits. Active women need walking room.

A-LINE — The A-line is an easy skirt to wear depending on the styling at the waistline. A high, round hip requires more darts or soft gathers. A tapered hip can wear a single dart or no dart as found in the typical wrap skirt. In order to camouflage a full thigh, the skirt's fullness should start above the hip line. Center front and back seams are slimming. The fullness in this skirt should harmonize with the style of the jacket. It goes best with the hipbone or hipline-length shaped jacket.

GORED, FLARED OR GATHERED — A gored skirt is a princess silhouette, and the same rules apply to seam spacing. Gored skirts fit in the waist and upper hip. *Four-, six-,* or *eight-* gored skirts are the most slimming and comfortable. Seams are slenderizing and enable the skirt to provide fullness at the most becoming place to camouflage large thighs. Six or eight gores allow adequate shaping for a high hip. A gored skirt with fullness at the hemline offers as much or more comfort and freedom than pants and is more becoming.

Flared skirts are better on the taller, slimmer figure, done in soft fabric. Short women (5′3″ [160 cm] or under) should avoid excessive flare at the hemline.

A very full gathered skirt is the least slimming. The softer the fabric, the more gathers you can get away with, however.

Hem Length

Your hem length should fall somewhere between your knee and your age.

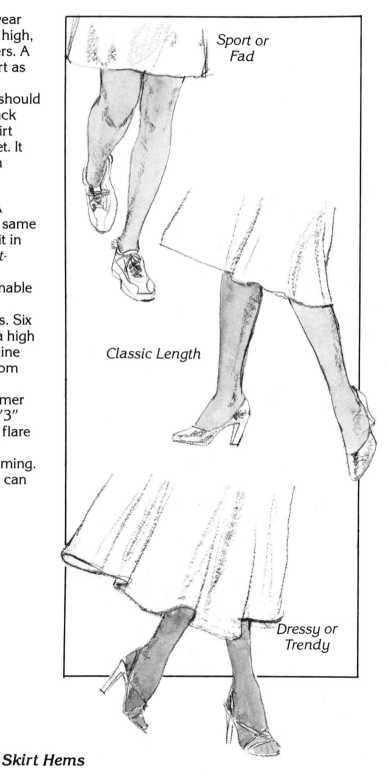

Sport or Fad

Classic Length

Dressy or Trendy

Skirt Hems

Skirts began to lengthen in the early 70s. Our eye is finally attuned to the longer length, although few women can wear their skirts as far down as fashion occasionally dictates. A well-dressed woman recognizes fashion but keeps her skirt lengths within the limits set by her own body.

Skirt lengths are variable and dependent upon the style of the garment, the hand of the fabric, the style of the shoe, and the shape and length of the leg. Most women have about three different skirt lengths in their wardrobes, which can be a problem when it comes to slips. The fashion-dictated mid-calf dress will make most women look dumpy. The trick is to reach a happy medium: skirts long enough to be fashionable, but short enough to look good.

Determining Length

The majority of your dresses and skirts will be worn at the most becoming point on your leg, and that is somewhere below the knee. Stand in front of a mirror and hold a skirt in front of your body. Right under the knee most legs get smaller, especially on the inside. That small area then shapes into the calf. The distance of the calf from the knee varies with the individual. Move the skirt up and down to determine how your leg looks with the skirt at different levels and with different shoes. You will find that with very high heels or a dainty shoe, the leg looks longer and you can get away with a longer skirt. A sturdy, heavy shoe with a lower heel calls for a shorter skirt which shows more leg.

The most becoming place on your leg is around one or two inches below the bottom of your knee. This is where you will wear most of your suits, skirts of heavier fabric, and daytime dresses. Measure the distance from the floor to the hemline in your stockinged feet. This is your basic skirt length.

If a dress is of a soft, drapey fabric or if it is an after-five or cocktail dress, the skirt can be a little longer. This type of dress should be worn with a daintier shoe. Examine your leg while wearing a delicate, strappy high-heeled shoe to discover how much longer you can go. Usually you will find that an inch or two longer will give you the fashionable feel without the dumpy look. Also, the taller you are and the thinner your calf, the longer you can wear your clothes.

If you are short or have thick ankles but yearn to wear a few long things, you should try a pair of classic boots with a moderate heel. Boots will camouflage a heavy leg, and because you will hem the garment to cover the top of the boot, the camouflage will be complete.

SHORT DRESSES — If you are a golfer and prefer to wear a skirt on the course, you should hem it at about knee length. Examine your knees. It will make a difference whether or not you plan to wear hose. Knees are not lovely, but hose help a lot. A young, firm knee could be completely exposed. A heavier knee will look better with the garment hemmed to the lower half of the knee.

Our motto has always been, "Show your knees if you please, but keep your thighs a surprise."

Low-heeled or flat shoes call for a skirt at the middle or bottom of the knee. Active sportswear is shorter than clothes for casual wear.

The periodic revival of the "Mini" or very short skirt is for the young, thin girl. For being young and lithe and cute, we find there is no substitute.

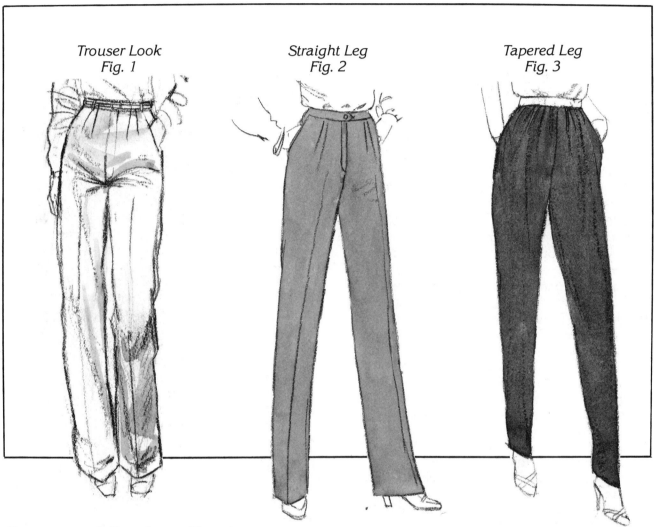

Trouser Look
Fig. 1

Straight Leg
Fig. 2

Tapered Leg
Fig. 3

Structural Design - Pants

Pants became accepted garments for females during World War II when women began working in war plants. The original patterns for ready-to-wear were merely adaptations of men's trousers, giving no thought to the differences of female anatomy. Fit has gradually improved, but it is still far from good in most makes. A good pair of slacks should be cut in the hip like a good straight skirt. This would allow the fabric to fall smoothly to the floor. Instead pants are often cut as if they were a flared skirt: the threads at the

center back and front seams join at an angle as if intended to flare at the thigh, and the threads of the fabric make a turn at the thigh level to enable the material to fall to the floor, causing wrinkles under the buttocks and excess fabric in the front groin (see Fig. 1).

When you purchase slacks, look for those which are cut in such a manner that the threads at the center front seam are parallel and the threads at the center back are almost parallel.

You will look thinner if your slacks are loose. You should be able to pinch about an inch of extra fabric on each side when standing. This amount of ease provides sitting room. If the fabric is stretchy there could be less ease, but avoid pants which are too tight.

There should be about one inch of room between your body and the fabric in the crotch. Insufficient ease in a crotch that is too high is uncomfortable and unattractive. Pants which ride up in the crotch so high as to make the contour of the genital region perfectly obvious are obscene. Women should start taking a closer look at themselves from the backside in their pants. It would come as a revelation to many women if they could view a motion picture of themselves walking in pants.

Slacks should be worn as long as possible without a break or fold above the shoe (see Fig. 2). They should barely skim the shoe in front and drop slightly in the back. The skimpier the leg, the shorter the pant must be. This fact gives added reason for choosing straight-leg pants.

Avoid cuffs. They flop when you walk and shorten your leg. Cuffs are a fad which surfaces from time to time.

The inset waistband rather than the elastic stretch variety gives a nicer finish to the waist so that you can tuck blouses in if desired (see Fig. 1).

Many figure faults can be camouflaged with pants which have the waistband designed to ride just below the waist instead of above it (see Fig. 2). The lowered, contoured waistband will hide a thick waist, camouflage a waistline which is too long or too short, and help to camouflage a round tummy. It is also more comfortable for those with a long crotch. The low waistband will not lift the pant on the body. A high hip or excess flesh around the waist can cause pants to ride up, causing discomfort and an unattractive crotch area.

We have rarely seen a pair of ready-to-wear pants which would not benefit from "tucking out" in the back. This alteration will eliminate the excess fabric found under the waistband in back and help eliminate some wrinkles under the buttocks and excess fabric in the front groin (see Alterations, Chapter 4, page 78).

Trouser pleats (Fig. 1 and 2), can be very becoming on the tapered hip with a slightly rounded tummy. The extra fullness in the groin de-emphasizes the thigh while the center front zipper fills in the hollow above the stomach. The result is a smoother, slimmer line.

The high hipped figure may want to change any pleats to several small tucks or gathers, depending on the fabric, to accommodate her high hip bones and high round tummy. The addition of a tie belt or buckle in the hollow of the waistline will help to de-emphasize the roundness of the stomach.

Fabric with drape is always more becoming. Recent fashion shows such fabric as crepe, jersey, soft cotton, silk and knits in pants. With softer fabrics the pants must offer more room in the hip area. We get the best of both worlds — soft fabric for slimming and more room for greater comfort. *Fashion-wise*, the main consideration is in the style of the leg. Flared and tapered pants fade in and out of fashion. Straight-leg pants are always in fashion because they are the most becoming (see Fig. 2).

A pair of pants should hang straight from the fullest part of the thigh. Any time a pant leg becomes more slender below the thigh, it will make the hips look bigger (see Fig. 3).

A moderate flare, especially if there is some shaping just above the knee, is very becoming (see Fig. 2). Never wear bell bottoms, however, if you already have one. The width of the pant leg at the bottom should relate to the foot size. A very skinny pant leg will make the foot appear large, and the reverse is true (see Fig. 3). A larger foot will appear in better balance if the pant leg is at least straight, allowing the hem to hang at the toe of the shoe rather than at the instep (see Fig. 2).

Never wear a girdle with pants. A girdle or tight panty hose give the monobuttock or "wasp behind" look. We prefer divisive splendor. If, for reasons of health, you must wear a girdle or support hose, wear your slacks looser.

JEANS — Jeans epitomize the generation gap in clothes. They require a young, slender body. The designer label has failed to improve the fit or look of even one middle-aged, overweight behind. If you feel you must wear jeans, choose those cut like slacks. Wear them a little looser and avoid a tight crotch.

JUMPSUITS — Jumpsuits are for young bodies. Jumpsuits, unless they are very loose and have at least one inch of distance between the body and the pant, will emphasize every figure flaw and add pounds. *Never* dance in a jumpsuit. The view from the rear is appalling!

PAJAMA & PALAZZO PANTS — Pajama and palazzo pants are most becoming because they are designed to flow like a skirt. They must be long enough in the crotch to not touch the body.

CULOTTES — Culottes are pushed to the masses on a three-year cycle. They never look as good as a skirt because ready-to-wear culottes are poorly fitted in the rear. However, they look good in front, especially if they have pleats or have wrap styling. Shop carefully to avoid the droopy, rump-sprung look in back.

SHORTS — There is a muscle on a woman's inner thigh which is a dead giveaway of her age when she wears shorts. It begins to sag about age 25, depending on how physically active she is.

Short shorts are for the very young. Jamaicas and Bermudas are more becoming. Knee-length or "city shorts" surface in fashion but never make it because only the young and the thin can carry off the look. Most women look ridiculous in knee-length shorts.

JACKETS WITH SLACKS — The best length for coats worn with pants is to the crotch in front. This gives the best balance between pants and coat. It also covers most of the bottom and all of the tummy.

If you are slender, you could wear a jacket which comes to the hip line. We never put a short jacket, to the hip bone or waist length, with pants on a mature body. Short jackets give brutal exposure to the tummy and the rear.

BLOUSES WITH SLACKS — Blouses with slacks are another matter. A long-sleeved blouse worn as an overblouse looks best worn between the hip bone and the hip line. There is a best length which will be uniquely yours. Have the overblouse long enough to nearly cover your tummy but short enough to show the groin, which is the slimmest part of the hip.

Generally, blouses look best when tucked into pants, especially when worn under a jacket or sweater.

SLEEVELESS OR SHORT-SLEEVED TOPS — Sleeveless or short-sleeved tops with slacks can be shorter. The sweatshirt types with a band can be a good camouflage for the tummy if they are loose enough to stay down over the hip bone.

A tucked-in blouse and a higher heel will make you look taller and slimmer. If you have a high tummy, you might consider wearing a scarf or self-belt tied in front to camouflage the roundness.

SHOES WITH PANTS — Because of your varied lifestyle you may need more pants to go with the different heel heights you wear for different occasions.

A good pant suit, the tailored variety that may be accessorized with hat and gloves, calls for a tailored, more covered-up, pant shoe with a medium heel. Lighter-weight, more casual summer pant sets, pant suits or dressy evening pants pair well with sandals. The height of the heel can be determined by comfort or fashion, but the pants must be hemmed to go with its own specific shoe.

Casual pants for work and play might be hemmed to go with a flatter, casual, comfortable shoe.

With all the help we can offer to make your pant life look better, we still feel that no matter how good you look in pants, you will look better in a skirt!

Applied Design - For Eye Appeal And Camouflage

Applied design is any device added to the structural design of a garment to make it more interesting, add style and personality or enable you to get in and out of it. Applied design can accentuate the positive and camouflage the negative.

Line can be very contradictory because your body may not be consistent.

☐ The shape of the face may be round or square, which would indicate a deep V, but the neck is long, which dictates a higher neckline. Fill in the V with a necklace or scarf.

☐ One might have a perfectly balanced oval face, with nice neck, shoulders and bustline but very wide hips. Applied design would be needed to broaded the shoulder in order to make the hips look narrower.

☐ A short neck might call for a deep V, but the figure also has narrow shoulders and a full bust which need shoulder broadening. Use yokes, collars or lapels.

We use applied design to balance the contradictions or to correct the architecture.

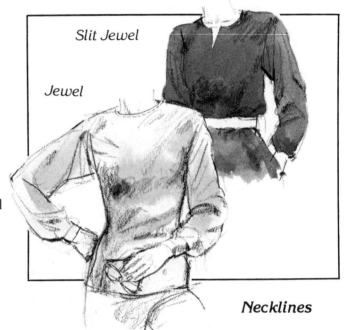

Slit Jewel

Jewel

Necklines

Necklines

Five factors should be considered in the choice of a neckline: width of shoulders, balance of the shoulders with the size of the bust, balance of the shoulders with the width of the hips, length of the neck and the shape of the face. In considering necklines, the concern is with the *width* and the *depth*. What does your body need and what will a given look do for it? How deep can you go and how wide can you go to achieve a balance with the figure as a whole? Horizontal lines broaden; vertical lines narrow.

Remember! We are primarily trying to balance the shoulders with the bust and the hips. The secret to line is *balance* and *proportion*.

Let us first consider necklines without collars.

JEWEL NECK — the jewel neck is considered an unfinished neckline. We add accessories and applied design, such as a slit, top stitching, embroidery, buttons, pins, necklaces or scarves, to help balance off the rest of the garment.

V-NECKS, SCOOPS, SQUARES (ALL COLLARLESS) — These neck shapes will accentuate face shape if repetitive, round shoulders, a head which is set forward, a dowager's hump, too long a neck, and poor posture. If you have any of these figure flaws you will need help when wearing collarless necklines. Use scarves, jewelry or an extra lay-on collar to balance the body or camouflage figure flaws.

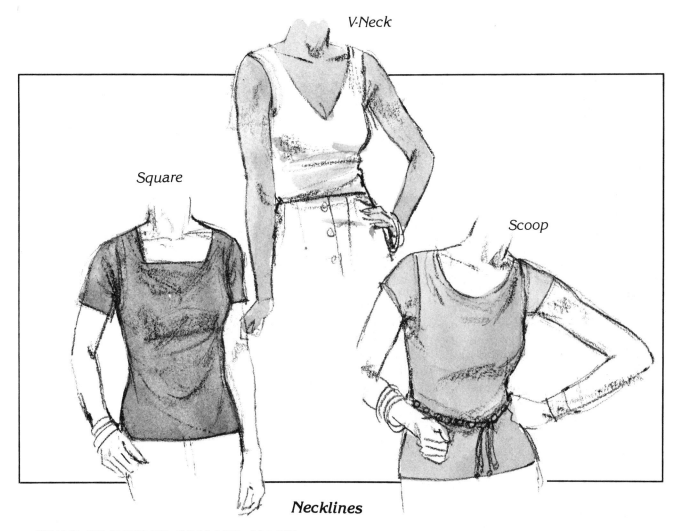

V-Neck

Square

Scoop

Necklines

STAND-UP BANDED COLLARS, MOCK TURTLES AND TURTLENECKS — A narrow stand-up banded collar can be worn by most figure types. Most people can wear mock turtlenecks unless the neck is extremely short or heavy. Turtlenecks are best on the medium to long neck. The choice of fabric is very important. More women can wear the thin, tissue knit or lightweight jersey fabric than can wear the bulky ribbed sweater knit or heavy fabric.

MANDARIN COLLARS — The stiff, straight-cut, true Mandarin collar looks best on the Oriental girl or on a dramatic-type woman.

COWL AND DRAPED NECKS — These depend on their width and depth for becomingness. The softer the fabric, the more body types can wear it. Large, full-busted women should be certain that the drape is placed above the bustline, not on it.

BOWS — The size and shape of bows tied at the neck vary with fashion. String ties and medium-sized bows can be worn by almost all body types, but the large, "pussycat" bows involve body type and personality. Soft fabric will fall softly without too much bulk, but firmer fabric adds bulk and width. Practice tying your bows to make them attractive.

If you have a long neck, try wrapping the ties around the neck for more sophistication instead of tying them into a bow.

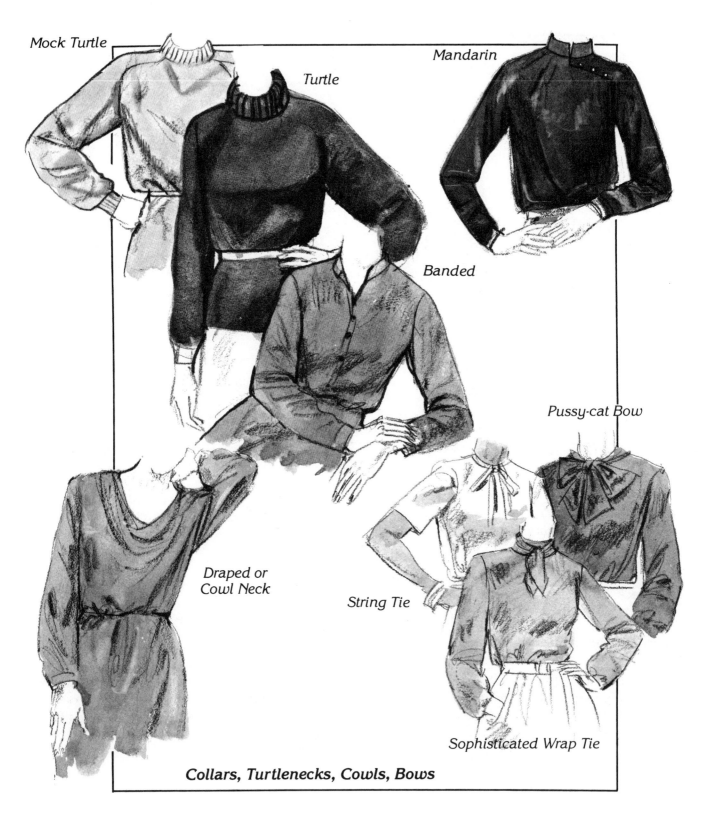

Mock Turtle

Turtle

Mandarin

Banded

Pussy-cat Bow

Draped or
Cowl Neck

String Tie

Sophisticated Wrap Tie

Collars, Turtlenecks, Cowls, Bows

COLLARS AND LAPELS — Collars and lapels must be scaled to your height and your size. Examine the lines of your collar to determine what the influence on shoulder width will be. A standard notched collar can be worn by all body types. Peaked collars tend to broaden and if not softened are masculine. Collars which point down can narrow the shoulder. Shawl collars which drape too deeply (to the waistline) can shorten the legs and look matronly.

If you have a forward-set head, or poor posture, collars set away from the neck in back are flattering. A thick or short neck will appear to be in better proportion if the collar is set away from the neck all around. Experiment with collar placement to achieve the best camouflage.

A dowager's hump benefits from a fuller collar in the back. (See page 51.)

Long, thin necks look good in collars with a high rise.

YOKES — Yokes which are high with no gathers below them have a broadening effect. The same yoke with gathers below it will not broaden. The gathers seem to have a softening effect on broad shoulders and yet a great balancing effect on narrow shoulders. Soft gathers below a yoke balance and camouflage a full bust. Yoke seaming which falls about midway down the arm's eye (armhole or sleeve seam) from the shoulder seems to be the most becoming. Shaped yokes in back are especially good on a broad shoulder to break the width. They are also good on the narrow shoulder.

SEAMS — Seams are slimming. "Easy-to-

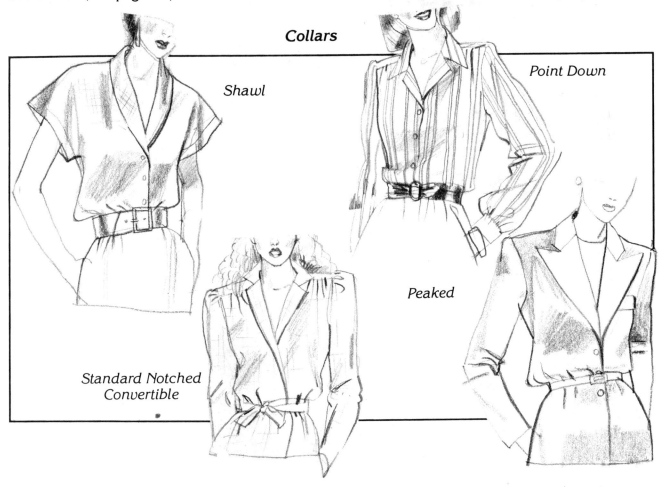

Collars

Shawl

Point Down

Standard Notched Convertible

Peaked

make" clothing which eliminates the seams will not look or fit as well as those garments which have seams and inset sleeves.

To Broaden The Shoulder

To make the shoulder look broader, use wider and shallower necklines, wider collars and lapels. Use yokes, off-center jewelry, scarves and horizontal top-stitching. Shoulder pads are helpful to the narrow shoulder.

To Narrow The Shoulder

To make the shoulder look narrower, use center interest such as buttons, bands, longer necklaces, scarves with center interest, narrower lapels, narrower and deeper necklines, and set-in sleeves.

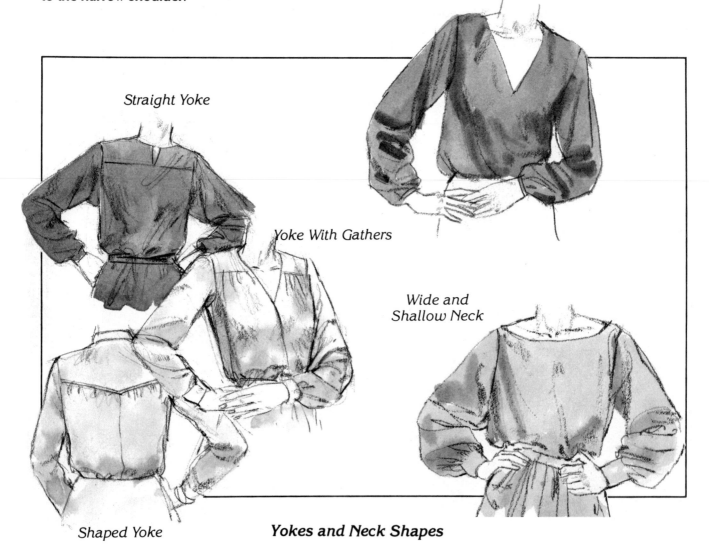

Straight Yoke

Yoke With Gathers

Shaped Yoke

Narrow and Deep Neck

Wide and Shallow Neck

Yokes and Neck Shapes

Sleeve Styles

Sleeves can be considered as both structural and applied design. The way in which the sleeve is attached to the garment could be considered structural design. The style, detail, fullness, etc., of the sleeve could be considered to be applied design.

SET-IN SLEEVES — The set-in sleeve is best on all body types. The seam of a set-in sleeve follows the crease or line which forms where the arm is connected to the shoulder. This sleeve type is the most youthful and gives balance to the body.

SLEEVE VARIATIONS — Whenever the stitching line of the sleeve or armhole varies from the natural crease line of the arm, you create problems unless you have perfectly proportioned shoulders.

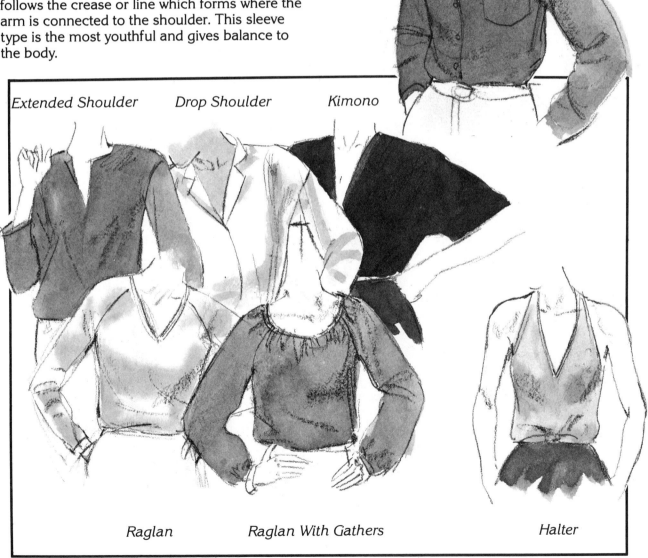

Set-in

Extended Shoulder   *Drop Shoulder*   *Kimono*

Raglan   *Raglan With Gathers*   *Halter*

1. A garment with the sleeve sewn just slightly farther out than the natural crease (extended shoulder) will make the shoulder look broader and the woman look matronly.

2. If the sleeve is sewn even farther out, as in a drop shoulder, it will accentuate any shoulder problem.

3. A raglan or dolman sleeve can be worn by those with perfectly proportioned shoulders which balance with the bust and the hip. These sleeve variations will make broad shoulders appear more broad and narrow shoulders appear more narrow. In the case of narrow shoulders and full bust, these styles will emphasize the bust, giving a pear shape to the upper body.

If a raglan sleeve is used in combination with gathers at the neck, however, the bad effect is diminished because the seam is lost in the gathers.

4. Only the well-proportioned shoulder with smooth flesh can wear a cut-back sleeveless garment or a halter neck. A halter neck will make a broad shoulder look huge and a narrow shoulder look smaller.

Sleeve Lengths

All body types can wear a *long slim* sleeve. Long sleeves are dressier and will go more places.

The ¾ *sleeve* is good on the well-proportioned arm of a medium to sturdy body with medium or small hands. If one has a slender wrist and large hands, the ¾ sleeve will make the hands appear to be very large. Tall girls must avoid the ¾ sleeve or they will appear to be growing out of their clothes. This rule does not apply to pushed-up sweater sleeves or rolled-up cuffs.

A *cap sleeve* will make the arm look fatter if the sleeve is tight. A heavy arm looks better in a

A *short sleeve* should reach to one inch (3 cm) below the crown of the bust. You must be very careful about sleeves which end near the elbow. Unless carefully styled, they can be very matronly.

cap sleeve which is loose. The cap sleeve is always better looking if it has a seam at the natural crease line of the arm and shoulder.

A *sleeveless* garment with the armhole cut in from the natural crease line will accentuate bony or fat shoulders and narrow shoulders. This is a particular problem with vests and boleros. The armhole must come to the natural crease line to look good. A sleeveless garment where the armhole ends slightly beyond the natural line can help to balance a narrow shoulder and a fat upper arm.

Sleeve Fullness

The fullness of a sleeve should always be scaled to your height and width. Everyone can wear a slim sleeve. The semi-full sleeve as found in cuffed blouses is also good on all body types. The full sleeve can add width, depending on the fabric. The fullness can start at the shoulder or it can flare out at the hip line.

The traditional puff sleeve is a young girl's look, seldom used by a fashionable, mature woman. It is seen in square dance dresses and costumes. It can broaden a narrow shoulder.

Released tucks or gathers at the shoulder line of a sleeve provide a good fashion look when done in very soft fabric. The look can broaden a narrow shoulder, but due to fickle fashion, it may date your garment.

Fullness in the hip area of a long sleeve should be avoided by those who have broad hips or who are short.

Pockets

The influence of pockets is determined by the direction of the lines of the design. The lines of the pocket and the placement on the garment should attract the eye to good features of the figure. Pockets which have vertical or slanted seaming are most graceful and will be more slimming. Patch pockets are the least slimming.

After solving your clothesline dilemma by applying these rules of good proportion, you may be feeling that all is lost. Do not despair, though; you may be able to salvage much of your current wardrobe by making simple alterations.

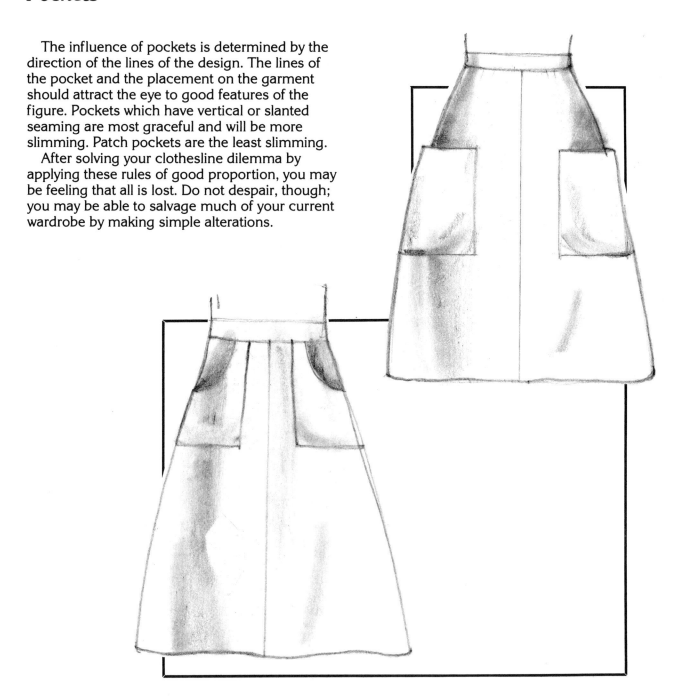

CHAPTER FOUR

Alterations And Fabric

RESCUING YOUR READY-TO-WEAR

Women desperately need to master basic sewing skills, if only to adjust ever-changing hemlines, repair poorly sewn ready-to-wear and make minor alterations. The ability to sew could ease your wardrobe budget. Much ready-to-wear could be greatly improved by utilizing some of the Fashion Academy's simple tricks of alteration.

Styling And Alteration For A High Hip

Hips generally fall into one of two categories which we described in Chapter 2, "Your Body Line," as high round (Fig. 1) or tapered (Fig. 2). Ready-to-wear clothes are shaped for tapered hips, which taper smoothly from waist to hip line. If there are any darts, they are stitched straight, permitting the size of the garment to expand in a gradual manner (Fig. 2a).

The presence of a high hip causes most garments to ride up, producing a fold of excess fabric just under the waistband all around. The garment is usually plenty big in the waist and lower hip but does not get big enough, high enough to accommodate the high hip, so it slides up on the body.

The high round hip looks best in clothes that have soft gathers which can release the needed fullness close to the waistline (Fig. 3a). Darts on this figure will work best if there are several small darts instead of the usual single large dart. The darts must be shaped to conform to the rounded body (Fig. 1a).

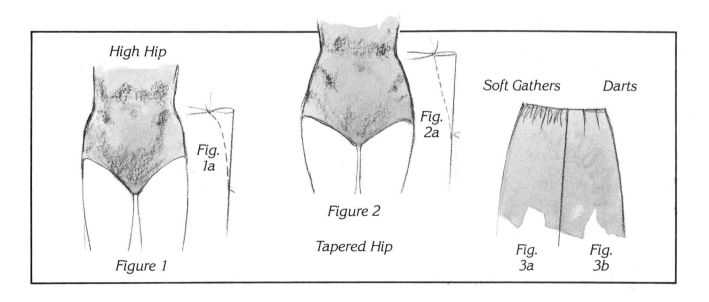

High Hip

Fig. 1a

Figure 1

Fig. 2a

Figure 2

Tapered Hip

Soft Gathers   Darts

Fig. 3a   Fig. 3b

The most effective way to alter ready-to-wear for a high hip is to change any darts to gathers. Sometimes this cannot be done, however, because the point of the dart has been marked with a small hole in the fabric.

To change darts to gathers, unpick the waistband or waistline seam for about two inches on each side of each dart. Unpick the dart. Stitch a row of long stitches on the waist seamline in the area of the dart. Then draw up the thread, causing the fabric to gather itself back to the original size. Adjust the gathers and restitch the waist seam (Fig. 3a).

If there is a hole in the fabric at the point of the dart, you can improve the fit by restitching the darts in a rounded shape to conform to the curve of the body (Fig. 1a). The ideal dart arrangement for a high hip is to divide a single dart into two small darts. Restitch the waistband or seam (Fig. 3b).

Even greater improvement is achieved if you can release, or let out, the side seams to allow addition of a second dart or put more fabric into the gathers.

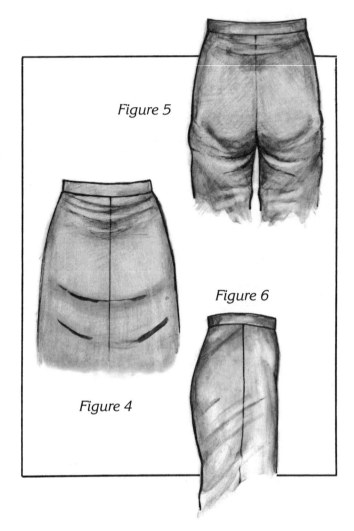

Figure 5

Figure 6

Figure 4

The Swayback Fitting Problem

If you have a high firm bottom, typical of the young figure, we might describe you as being "swayback." It is not a derogatory term, but merely a way of describing the hollow above a shapely derriere. This figure looks good in pants, but fitting can be a problem because of the roll of fabric which appears just under the waistband in the back. This roll of fabric will also occur in skirts (Fig. 4). This figure will usually have excessive wrinkles below the buttocks in pants as described below and as shown in Figure 5. The wrinkles act as arrows pointing to the thigh and causing a ripple on the side in the thigh area, accentuating any fullness there. The excess fabric can be removed at the waistline, greatly improving the appearance of the garment.

The Flat Bottom Fitting Problem

As the human body ages, there is a natural tendency for the tissue to respond to the pull of gravity. This is most apparent in the hip area. When the bottom drops, the figure flattens in back. Meanwhile on the side back, the dropping flesh creates a hollow, which accentuates any bulge in the thigh area. A woman who may have had very flat thighs when young may develop a bulge as she matures. This problem is emphasized by ill-fitting skirts and pants.

The flat bottom looks good in skirts and can look good in pants if they are fitted fairly loose and are styled in a straight cut. Ready-to-wear assumes that all women have rounded behinds. If there is no fullness on the body, the fabric droops below the buttocks in back, causing skirts to appear "rump sprung" or look longer in back (Fig. 6). Pants will have wrinkles under the buttocks which extend toward the thigh on the side, exaggerating any bulge (Fig. 5). The excess fabric needs to be removed at the top, an act that will lift the garment and allow the skirt or pant to hang properly in the back.

Alteration For Swayback, Flat Bottom

The remedy for both problems — the swayback and the flat bottom — is the same. With the garment on, pin a tuck in the fabric just under the waistband. This will take out the wrinkles of the swayback figure or lift the fabric to the proper level over the flat rear or under the buttocks. Unpick the stitching and remove the waistband across the back of the garment. Trim off the amount of fabric you had in the tuck. The amount which needs to be trimmed off could

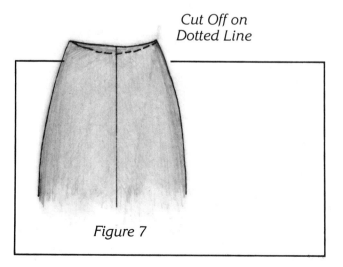

Cut Off on Dotted Line

Figure 7

vary from ½ inch (1.3 cm) to 1 inch (2.5 cm) at the center back and taper to nothing at the side seams (Fig. 7). Restitch the waistband in place. In pants this will shorten the crotch, so it is necessary to have adequate crotch length to allow for the tuck.

If this alteration produces a better fit, you will find that it will be standard procedure for all your skirts, dresses and pants, because your body does not conform to the image clothing manufacturers have of how a human body is shaped. Because most women need the correction, it is obvious the cutters are in error. Now that you can visualize your fitting needs and provide solutions to some of your problems you are ready to sharpen up your expertise in the fabric department.

Fashion And Fabric In Garment Design

Fashion begins with fabric. They are inseparable. *Your fashion sense will develop only as fast as your fabric sense* and no faster. The creator of fine clothing is an artist who works with cloth. The degree of success depends upon the skill with which the artist combines fabric and design.

Fabric will speak to you if you will become sensitive to its message. Observation is your best tool in furthering your understanding of fabric. Whenever you see clothing which meets your approval, whether in a store, on a friend, or in an advertisement, try to discern what the fabric might be and what characteristic makes it suitable for the particular garment in which it is used.

In describing or working with fabric, four factors are involved: *hand, fabric design, fiber* and *weave.*

Hand describes the way the fabric drapes, its texture or feel. In addition, when we say that a fabric of quality has a good hand, we mean that you can *feel* the quality, or that the fabric will work well in the making of a garment. The hand of the fabric is the primary factor determining pattern selection or the design of the garment. It is the single most important element determining success in use of fabric. Additional knowledge of the other factors will enhance your enjoyment of fabric, but an understanding of hand is imperative.

Fabric design or *pattern in cloth* is achieved in myriad ways: in the weave, the texture of the yarn, its bulk or fineness, space dying of yarn, printing of the finished cloth, applique, embroidery, etc. The list is endless. The design of the cloth will greatly influence the choice of pattern or the design of the garment.

Fiber is the filament or staple from which yarn is spun and then knitted or woven into a textile. Fabric fiber might be of natural, man-made or synthetic origin, or a blend of two or more. The finished fabric can be of no better quality than the fiber of which it was made. Good fiber, on the other hand, can be destroyed by poor manufacturing and finishing processes.

Weave describes the method used to interlace yarn into fabric. It might be a simple process, as in a plain weave, or it might be a very complicated one, as in a jacquard. The same type of weave in different fibers will have a different name. For example, a twill weave in a cotton is denim, in a wool it is gabardine, and in a silk, surah.

Natural Fibers Versus Synthetics

When synthetic fabrics burst on the market, beginning with nylon hosiery in the '40s, there began a national switch towards man-made fabrics in the United States. American women acquired, with dubious pride, the title "Polyester Princesses." The pendulum has now started to swing back with greater demand for natural fibers. Each type of fabric has advantages and

problems. You must decide which best suits your lifestyle, your physical requirements, your taste and your budget. The most common of the natural fibers are cotton, silk, wool and linen.

The first of the man-made fabrics (not a true synthetic, inasmuch as it has a cellulose base similar to cotton) was rayon, which offers almost as much comfort as a natural fabric. Rayon and its descendants, acetate and tri-acetate, tend to wrinkle and ravel when used by themselves, but offer miraculous wrinkle resistance when used in a blend with other fibers. The true synthetics, made of petroleum derivitives, are nylon, polyester and acrylic (orlon).

It is no accident that designers use fabrics made of natural fibers in their clothes. Fabric of natural fibers has a richer look and can be molded into a design or made to conform to body curves more readily than fabric of synthetics.

Any woman who has owned a silk blouse or dress can attest to the elegantly feminine feeling one gets from wearing silk. A good wool suit or coat spoils us for polyester. Pure cotton clothing makes hot weather bearable. Good wool sheds wrinkles, gives warmth without weight and wears for years without losing its shape. Natural fabrics allow passage of air, absorb perspiration and allow it to evaporate. Natural fiber fabrics can be altered, hems changed, seams let out; synthetics cannot, since they suffer from abrasion at seams and edges. Natural fabrics do wrinkle, but a few creases are less worrisome, it seems, when we know they are expensive wrinkles!

Polyester and nylon are susceptible to perspiration odor and grease stains which can be almost impossible to wash out. Try a vinegar rinse on perspiration stains, a pre-spotting solution for grease stains, and for ball point pen marks, soak with hair spray before washing.

Generally you will get more elegance, comfort and longevity from natural fibers. Synthetics offer washability and wrinkle resistance. With blends you could get the best of both worlds.

If you wear synthetic fabrics, spend extra to acquire those which *look* like natural fiber fabrics. Choose, for example, polyester crepe de

Chine which *looks* like silk, Rayon-polyester which *looks* like real linen, nylon jersey which *looks* like silk jersey, and acrylic which *looks* like wool.

Synthetic fibers will not, as a rule, dye clear, bright intense colors. A black synthetic fabric appears gray next to a black silk or wool. Of the synthetics, acrylic accepts bright dyes most successfully but acrylic washes less well than other man-made fabrics and has a tendency to develop tiny balls of fuzz or to "pill." Winter is known as the expensive season because the rich Winter colors are usually found only in expensive natural fabric — silks, wools and pure cotton.

Clothing Design

Design in relation to clothing can be divided into two categories: Structural and applied. Structural design refers to the shape controllers — seams, darts, etc., Applied design refers to collars, cuffs, pockets, buttons, belts, top-stitching, etc.

You have clothes in your closet which you never wear. The most common problem with them is poor fit, and this is the only fault which has nothing to do with fabric. Analyze your clothes and try to determine what their problems are. Here are some possibilities:

□ You might find that the color, texture or hand of the fabric is unsuitable for your season, figure or personality.

□ Perhaps the hand of the fabric or the design of the fabric is unsuitable for the design of your garment.

□ Another common fault is that the design of the garment is not suitable for your figure type or your personality.

Choose fabric to go with your garment design:

□ *Interesting fabric* requires a pattern with little applied design. The more interesting the fabric, the simpler the pattern should be.

□ *Simple fabric* can take more intricate patterns and often needs applied design (top-stitching, etc.) to bring out the beauty of the fabric.

□ *Soft, drapey fabric* can take a design with few seams or darts and still give the illusion of a form-fitting garment. Soft fabric is slenderizing. Drapey fabrics do not make up well in patterns with much structural detail or applied design.

□ *Crisp fabrics* require seams and shape controllers to give form to the garment. Crisp fabrics are less slenderizing.

The becomingness of fabric is influenced by:

□ *Texture* — Bulky fabrics increase size; they tend to enlarge the heavy figure and engulf the petite figure.

□ *Light reflection* — Shiny fabrics reflect light and increase size. Shiny fabrics compete with sleekness of hair and smoothness of skin. Dull, light-absorbing fabrics decrease size and act as a foil for the skin and hair, making them appear more shiny.

□ *Crispness or Stiffness* — Stiff fabrics increase size. Soft fabrics decrease size and they drape gently over body curves. (The possible exception to this is silk jersey, which shows every roll and bulge.)

□ *Transparency* — Transparent fabrics usually must be used in great quantity, so they tend to increase size. (Silk chiffon, due to its soft hand, is an exception.)

□ *Color* — The eye goes to the lightest part of the costume. Light colors are less slenderizing.

In summary, then, we could say that a becoming fabric is low in bulk, light-absorbing, opaque, soft, drapable and a becoming color. This type of fabric is also easier to sew.

Choosing A Print

Choice of the appropriate fabric print largely influences the success of a garment. The design or print of the fabric can contribute to or detract from a garment's appearance. The visual effect of a fabric is influenced by the hand or drape of the fabric, its texture, design and color. On a printed fabric, the design is the overall pattern created by the compilation of individual motifs. A motif is one unit of a design. Motifs are classified according to style as geometric, realistic, stylized or abstract. A few facts and cautions relating to each season might prove helpful in choosing your fabric.

Winter colors present the most difficulty in obtaining an attractive print. Winters will have more success with natural fibers in expensive fabrics. Winter colors lend themselves particularly well to geometric and abstract print motifs.

Summers will have no problem in finding good prints in any style.

Spring colors are particularly suited to stylized florals.

Autumn colors fall comfortably into leafy, earthy, stylized or abstract prints.

In any print, the colors of your season should dominate. Colors of other seasons may be present to add interest, but they should be included only in small amounts. You must be able to wear your own accessories with the print, and you should not have to alter your cosmetic colors. Prints should be chosen to enhance and define your personality. Keep in mind that soft, muted, curving lines in prints are more Yin, and straight, distinct, severe lines are more Yang.

GEOMETRIC MOTIFS — Geometrics include plaids, checks, stripes and circles. They are acceptable for any personality. A geometric is good to use providing you consider the size or scale of the motif in relation to the wearer. Always hold the fabric against your body in front of a mirror to see if the geometric is going to wear you — an especially risky possibility with plaids of great color contrast and considerable size. Small geometrics can blend into a blur from a distance and appear to change color. A red and white check, for instance, viewed from a distance may appear to be pink. Always observe fabric from a distance.

Stripes of strong color contrast and equal size waver and shimmer. They are disconcerting to sew. Tiny polka dots might make a good blouse but a dull dress. Large geometrics are generally safe in a blouse or a long skirt, but they are dangerous in a street-length dress unless the woman is very tall. In linear geometrics, the structural line of the garment should be angular

rather than curved to harmonize the fabric design. Plaids generally sew up poorly in a princess line. Plaids are never slimming, but they will not enlarge your figure if they are of a smaller scale and moderate color contrast.

Plaids accentuate broad, square shoulders, unless used on the bias. In general, plaids are best used for skirts or slacks in muted colors.

As a general rule, irregular stripes (those not close together and of unequal size and spacing) are more interesting and more slimming if worn horizontally because the eye is led to cross the stripe by the variation of space, color, etc.

REALISTIC MOTIFS — Realistic prints attempt to duplicate natural or man-made objects. They include flowers which look as if they are still on the plant, animals from a zoo, or any object that is drawn to give an accurate portrayal of the actual object. They are fun in children's clothes, on quilts, furniture or crafts. But realistic motifs often show little imagination on the part of the designer and can become boring and monotonous. Children love them, however.

Consideration must be given to the location of seams when making a garment from a realistic print because you can't cut through a cow or a rose with impunity. Generally speaking, we do not recommend realistic prints for adult garments with the exception of fun wear.

STYLIZED MOTIFS — Stylized motifs represent an artist's impression of a flower, animal or man-made object. They show imagination, and the designs are well suited to clothing because the art is one-dimensional in keeping with the flat fabric. Observe the same rule of scale as with geometric motifs. A stylized print is usually not disturbed by seaming because the motif does not pretend to be a real thing. The stylized prints are often done in very tiny motifs and can be too busy or matronly in a street-length dress. Be cautious of those which might resemble a print found in night wear if you are making a day dress. Consider the tiny ones more for blouses. Beware of stylized prints which include too many colors; they can blend into a dusty blur when viewed from a distance. Stylized prints seem to be the most common of all fabric print designs. Perhaps this is why it is so difficult to find a good one. Prints of medium size, clear harmonizing colors and not too many different hues are the most attractive. Muted colors are also good if they harmonize and look good to you when viewed from a distance.

ABSTRACT MOTIFS — Abstract prints are splashes of form and color. They are very pleasing in fabric design and are often quite sophisticated in feeling. We often find abstracts of geometric or stylized designs. Observe the rule of scale and choose a pattern in which the seams harmonize with the print — curved seams with curvy lines and architectured seaming with straight lines. Try to choose prints on which the motifs are spaced in such a way as not to require matching. Working with some of the weird ones can be a time-consuming and frustrating experience. If the motif is wavy or random, it may be impossible to match. If such is the case, recognize that you have reached the limitation of your fabric, and cease to worry about it. Some abstract prints are so large or so extreme that they are suitable only for at-home lounge wear or as a wall decoration.

If you are shopping for fabric and see a print, it should say something to you, such as "I would make a great day dress, or a good pant set, or a play dress for four-year-old Susie." If it doesn't speak, don't buy it, even if it is pretty.

Always unfold the bolt, stand in front of a mirror and drape the fabric over your body for the full length of the intended garment, then observe the effect. Is the color becoming? Will it make up in your pattern? Are you wearing the print or is it wearing you? Will it go with your present accessories? Will it need a trim to raise it out of the ordinary — and if so, is the trim available without weeks of looking?

Be more observant of ready-to-wear garments and the fabrics used in the ones you like. Do more looking and less buying. Never stockpile a fabric without attaching a note reporting what it "said" and why you bought it. That fabric may never speak again!

Care And Cleaning Of Your Wearables

An American woman interprets "Washable" to mean, "Throw it in the washing machine." She allows the load to agitate a full 14 minutes because that is the maximum time on her machine. If you have towels which are frayed on the selvedge while the centers are intact, you are wearing out your clothes in the washer. For most of your garments, pre-treat spots and soiled areas, then agitate no more than eight minutes in warm water. Wash your dainty belongings by hand. Plain colored silk blouses can usually be hand washed. Wrap immediately in a towel, wait 15 to 30 minutes and press on the wrong side with a warm iron. It takes about 30 minutes to iron a silk blouse, but if you have any skill at all, your blouse will look even better than when it comes from the dry cleaners.

Fabrics shrink when subjected to moisture, heat and agitation at the same time. Inefficient dry cleaning equipment can result in an excess of moisture in the cleaning solution causing shrinkage. Too rapid or too hot drying cycles at the dry cleaners can also shrink a garment, even one which has been cleaned many times previously.

Polyester suits which may have lost their spark from wear or washing, can sometimes be revived by a trip to a good dry cleaner. Your cleaner can remove some stains which have defied your efforts and a good professional press can perk up a limp and lazy garment.

Use care in selection of a dry cleaning establishment. Brush, spot-clean, air out and protect your good clothes from soil. Even the best dry cleaning is hard on fabric.

Keep your clothes clean and in good repair. Good organization in this part of your life helps everything else to run more smoothly.

Using the information you have on color, line, lifestyle and fabric selection, you now can begin the exciting adventure of discovering your personality.

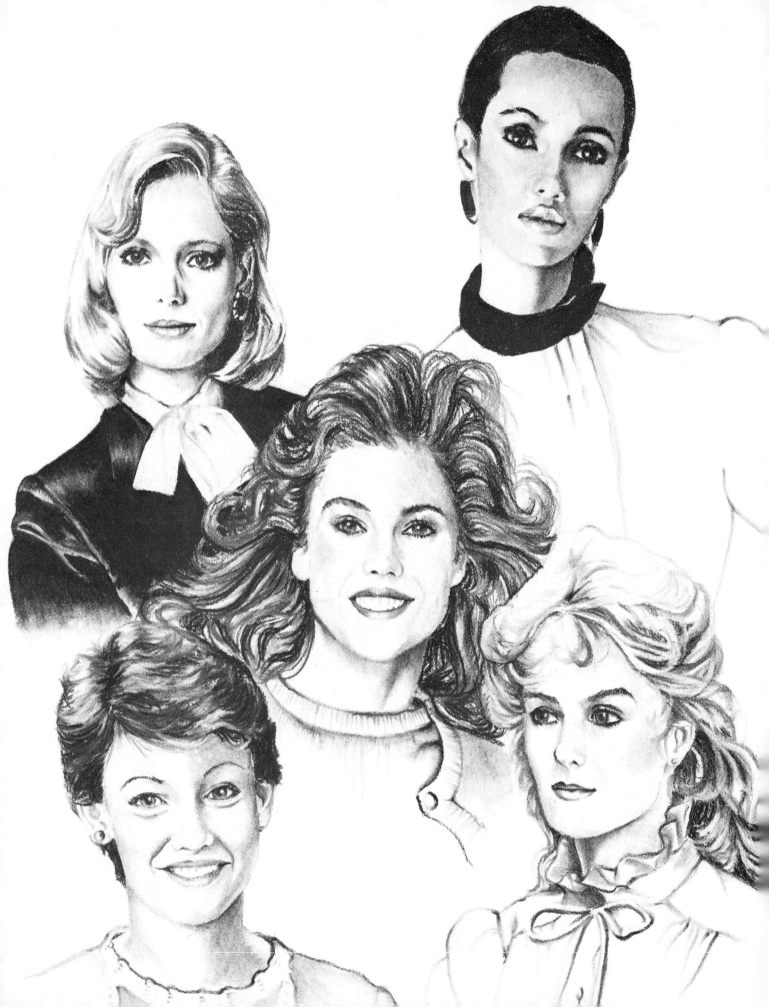

CHAPTER FIVE

Personality
YOUR INDIVIDUAL CHARM

Every woman is unique. Discovering who you are and how to develop your own image is the purpose of this chapter.

The personality we are considering is the personality of appearance: the way people see you, how you look to the world. Your coloring, your bone structure, your nervous system, muscle tone, adipose tissue and environment all determine your personality. The first four are inherited and cannot be changed. You cannot move your bones around, for example. You are who you are. But adipose tissue, which is fat, can be changed. Environment can be changed. Your environment as a child largely shaped the person you are today, but the way you looked also helped to shape your environment. A delicate blonde child is treated differently than a wiry brunette child. If you were the tallest girl in your school when you were in the third grade, it had an impact on your personality. You may never have adjusted to the fact that the rest of the girls have caught up with you and you are actually an average-sized woman, perhaps with a slender bone structure. Many people try to change themselves but end up a poor imitation. We could dress you up to be any personality we wanted and you might get away with it if you didn't move or open your mouth. As soon as you moved or spoke, however, you'd give yourself away. You cannot change your muscle tone or nervous system which control the way you move and react to stimuli. Redheads, blondes and brunettes, for example, have characteristic personalities because they grew up with those colorings and have been treated accordingly. You've heard that blondes have more fun? They

do — because they appear guileless. If you don't think people react differently to different colorings, think, if you will, when you ever saw a picture of a blonde devil or a brunette angel. We have been subconsciously preconditioned to respond in certain ways toward certain types of appearance.

You have discovered your season and found which colors look best on you. You have examined your body proportion and decided how best to use line and design. You are now going to analyze your personality and discover how to dress in harmony with it. When you really understand your colors, your line and your personality and know how to relate the three to clothing selection, you have *personal style.*

If you are fortunate, you might number among your acquaintances one or two women who have personal style. A woman who has it always looks good. She consistently dresses in keeping with her total personality and lifestyle. The woman who manages to get herself together for a big party once a year or for her bridge club meeting every month does not deserve much credit. It is the woman who always looks good no matter where you see her — shopping at the grocery store, watering her lawn, browsing at the shopping mall — who deserves applause. She is not always dressed up, but she is dressed in the best garment of its kind for whatever activity in which she is engaged. Her house might catch fire in the middle of the night. The press comes to take a picture and there she stands, holding the hose, in her nightgown — the right color, the right line and the right personality. She has personal style!

Yang and Yin Theory of Contrasts

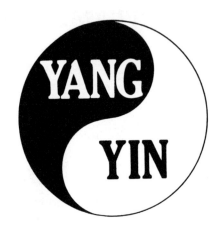

Yang	Yin
Dark	Light
Sun	Moon
Oak tree	Vine
Masculine	Feminine
Dark hair or complexion	Light hair or complexion
Large (bones or facial features)	Small (bones or facial features)
Strong and sturdy	Fragile and delicate
Mature	Youthful
Sophisticated	Unsophisticated
Independent	Dependent
Conservative	Flamboyant
Pragmatic	Artistic
Deliberate	Spontaneous
Do-it-yourselfer	Hire-it-done
Firm.	Tender.

It is a talent; it is an art. Some are born with it, others have to work to acquire it.

This is a fun concept. You might learn to understand and appreciate yourself, your husband, your children, loved ones and maybe even your neighbor.

In describing people, there are so many words with unfortunate connotations that we needed to establish a vernacular that would have less chance of offending our students. Men and women have both feminine and masculine qualities. Our society, however, has made us wary of being labeled with these terms. Men have qualities of gentleness, tenderness and nurturing. Women have qualities of independence, assertiveness and strength. Women don't like to be told they are masculine any more than men like to hear they have feminine traits. Adapting the symbol of Yin and Yang enabled us to evaluate the human qualities of an individual without threatening the ego.

The Yin and Yang symbol, found in all Oriental cultures, represents the balance between the contrasts found in the universe.

We have chosen six personality classifications first suggested by Harriet McJimsey in her book *Art In Clothing Selection* (Harper & Row). Ms. McJimsey used "athletic" for one of her classifications. We found, however, that the word "athletic" conjured up visions of smelly gym socks and offended some women so classified because they didn't want to be identified as jocks. So we changed this classification to "natural," a term that carries much more positive connotations.

The six personality classifications are: Dramatic, Natural, Classic, Romantic, Gamin and Ingenue.

YIN AND YANG PERSONALITY RELATIVITY

— Dramatic and Natural are the most Yang because of their taller or sturdier body structure and stronger facial features.

Gamin and Ingenue are the most Yin because they are small and youthful looking.

Classic and Romantic are both feminine and mature personalities. Classic is more sophisticated and controlled, while Romantic is more flamboyant.

To help you understand who you are, let us go back in memory to your childhood and discover how you became what you are today.

Children are small and as such are all Yin. For purposes of understanding yourself, however, we will start thinking about children in the same way as the women they become. The small Gamin, being more masculine, we will consider as Yang, and the small Ingenue, being more feminine, we will consider as Yin.

You were a combination of the two, but one was dominant. The dominance of your Yin side and your Yang side will change at different periods of your life. Which little girl were you?

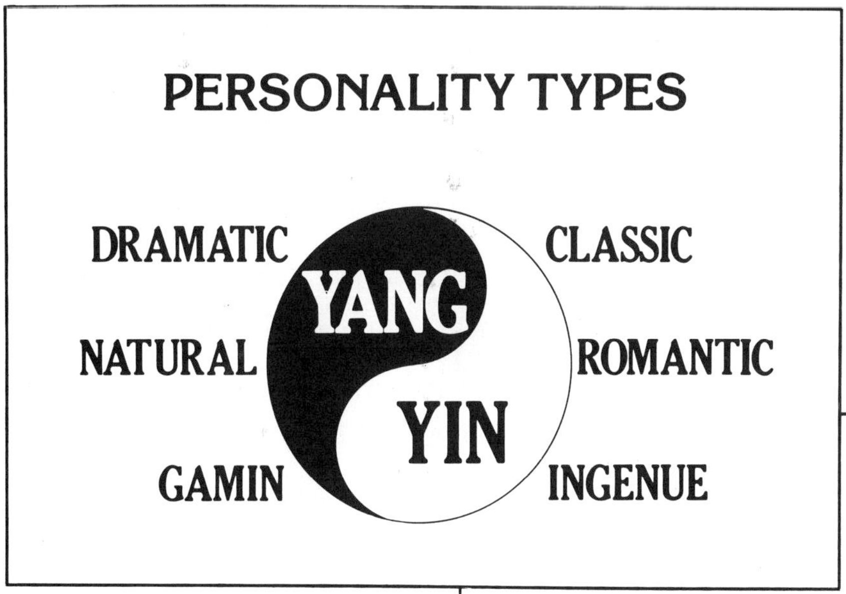

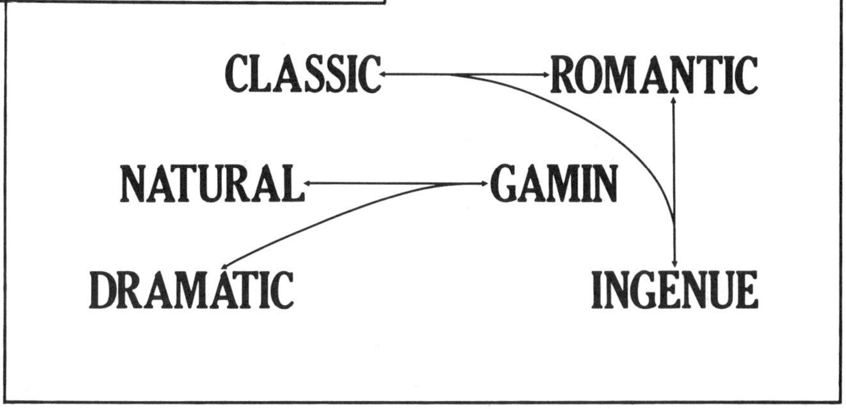

PERSONALITY TYPES

DRAMATIC   **YANG**   CLASSIC

NATURAL   ROMANTIC

GAMIN   **YIN**   INGENUE

CLASSIC———ROMANTIC

NATURAL———GAMIN

DRAMATIC   INGENUE

INGENUE — THE MOST YIN — The Ingenue is more likely to be dependent on other people for assistance or security. The Ingenue is small-boned and delicate, a feminine little lady. Often chubby because she is a more sedentary type, she likes dresses and usually stays clean. She loves dolls and likes to play house. Moody, manipulative and dumb like a fox, she pouts when she doesn't get her way, and someone always helps her to lift, carry and repair.

GAMIN — THE MOST YANG — The Gamin is independent. She never gets lost in a store — Mother gets lost. She is a small, wiry tomboy who loves jeans and boys' sports. The Gamin moves quickly, scuffs her shoes, takes tumbles and gets dirty. Impulsive, she flares up if she gets mad, but then it is over. She is impatient, can fix anything and would rather do a project herself.

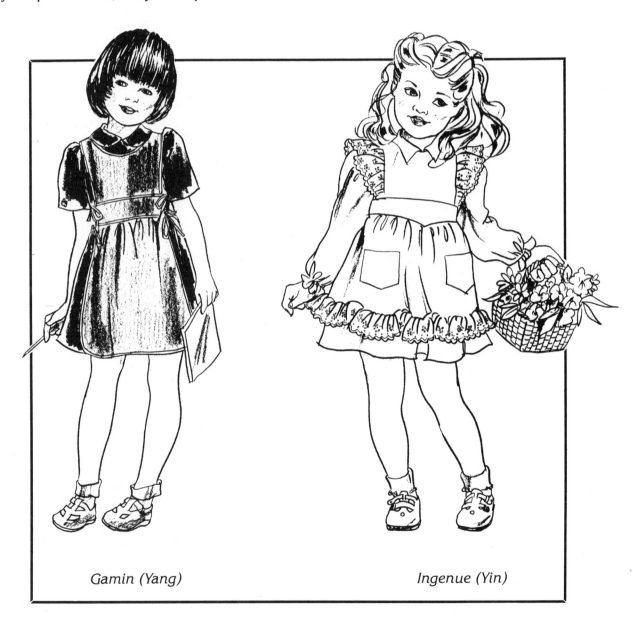

Gamin (Yang)

Ingenue (Yin)

As these two personalities mature they show contrasting characteristics. An Ingenue will cry first, then get mad. A Gamin gets mad first, then cries. An Ingenue cries beautiful tears, melting every heart. A Gamin bawls, with red eyes and a stuffed-up, runny nose. The Ingenue's grass could be knee-high, but she would never mow it. She would not wash a car, paint a wall or repair a light fixture. She has all the patience in the world —she knows that if she waits long enough, someone will do the job for her.

The Gamin is impatient. She mows her own lawn, paints her own walls, changes her own tires and fixes her own appliances because no one can do the job fast enough or good enough to suit her.

If you were to punish these two little girls by sending them to their rooms, the Gamin would beg not to be isolated. Being alone is torture for her because she likes to be where the action is. The Ingenue would stomp off, sulking, with revenge on her little mind. Two weeks later Mother would find crayon on the wall, under the drape. The Ingenue would swear, "I never did it!" The Gamin might write on the wall but if Mother didn't notice her artwork, the Gamin would call attention to it. She would rather face the consequences now and get them over with.

Give an Ingenue a list and she will do it. Give a Gamin a list and she will lose it.

When stealing chocolate chips, the Gamin will rip open the bag, spill the chips on the floor and smear the chocolate on her face and clothing. Gamins cannot lie because the evidence is always obvious. An Ingenue will make a delicate hole in the bottom, slip out a few pieces of chocolate and replace the bag precisely where she found it, leaving no trace. She will look you squarely in the eye and say, "I didn't do it!"

In grammar school, the Gamin usually gets the blame for what the Ingenue does.

We are all a combination of Gamin and Ingenue, but one will dominate. Your place in the family, the sex of your siblings, where you lived, the personality of your parents — all had influence in developing your personality. It may be helpful to imagine how you might have developed under different influences.

Regardless of how Gamin you might have been, however, there will be an emergence of the Ingenue at about age 40. Some call it menopause madness, mid-life crisis, a passage, or tired blood. Whatever you call it, your family may think you have flipped the day you refuse to fix your 12-year-old a peanut butter sandwich and suggest he make his own and one for you, too.

Which small girl were you, and how did your Gamin and Ingenue sides mature?

As each of us matures there must be a balance of Yin and Yang in the personality. There is always a balance in the well-adjusted, mature person. We see an imbalance in the woman's libber and in the male chauvinist. Both are maladjusted and threatened. They go around with a chip on their shoulder, begging someone to knock it off so that they can attack with the pent-up energy of their frustrations.

The Dramatic and Natural, which are Yang personalities, matured from the little Gamin, your Yang side.

The Romantic and Classic personalities matured from the small Ingenue, your Yin side.

You can stay Gamin your whole life, providing you remain short and your facial features small. Your Ingenue side should mature into a Classic or a Romantic. There are, however, some 40-year-old Ingenues running around trying to look and act like their teen-age daughters in a vain attempt to recapture their youth.

Study the Personality Analysis Chart on pages 100 and 101. Determine which personality or which combination of personalities most nearly describes you. After you have decided, have a family member or friend read it and give their opinion.

It is possible to have a combination of Yin features and a Yang body or vice versa. A good example of this dichotomy was Hoss Cartwright (the late actor Dan Blocker) of the "Bonanza" TV show. He had a large Yang body and a Yin baby face. His big, blue eyes and light coloring softened his Yang body.

Al Pacino of the movie "The Godfather" has a short Yin body and a strong, sophisticated Yang face with dark coloring. Dark coloring always adds sophistication and is Yang. Light coloring appears more innocent and is Yin.

This contrast is obvious in some Oriental women who have petite Yin bodies and large, dramatic facial features which are Yang. Think of

the six personalities as forming a continuum stretching from the extreme Yin to the extreme Yang. Your own personality will fall somewhere along the line. Your position on the continuum will vary at different times of your life and could take a different turn in the space of one day. You could be a Natural all day — gardening, playing tennis and washing your car. By evening, in contrast, you put some curl in your hair, add false eyelashes, put on a soft, feminine dress and become a Romantic. You can have the best of both worlds.

The two personalities which cannot be combined in one woman are the Dramatic and

CONTINUUM OF PERSONALITY

YANG   *YIN*

the Ingenue, because they are opposites. You could not take a Debbie Reynolds and make a Cher Bono out of her.

Life situations and circumstances may push us one way or another, but eventually the real you will surface.

You may have been the boy your father never had. You may have been the oldest girl of a large family or the youngest little darling of a mother who loved ribbons and bows. Or you might be the wife of an Ingenue man (though we would hesitate to tell a man he was an Ingenue).

Just for fun, let's take a look at some examples of personality types in action.

Two Ingenues got married and sat in bed their whole wedding night waiting for someone to get up and turn off the light.

Two sisters went off to Vassar College with the smaller Autumn Gamin carrying the six-foot Spring Ingenue's suitcase.

The kitchen water pipe burst, leaving the Winter Gamin bride, the plumber and the mother-in-law frantically trying to stem the flow and mop up. The Spring Ingenue spouse arrived home, surveyed the pandemonium and asked, "How soon can we have dinner?"

The 180-pound statuesque Natural-Classic Summer Ingenue capably ran a large corporation, then went home to a Classic husband who washed her windows, took care of her car and helped with the dishes because he knew she was not capable of managing alone.

All of the personalities are intriguing.

The Dramatic is the model type. No one has to teach a Dramatic how to walk; she was born with a slither.

The Natural is always covered with mysterious bruises, but she can never recall bouncing off walls or bumping into the furniture. She needs to avoid gum-soled shoes — she moves so fast the sticky soles can't keep up. Naturals have scuffed-up shoes and snags in their hosiery. They are open and honest and may suffer from foot-in-mouth disease.

The Classic is softly sophisticated. One cannot imagine a Classic being awkward, ungracious or impolite. She is in control of herself and the situation. The Classic cries alone.

The Romantic is born possessing feminine wiles. She wiggles when she walks and she giggles when she talks. Men love her — she seems so helpless.

The coloring of a Romantic often has some effect on her personality. If a blonde, Spring Romantic such as Zsa Zsa Gabor were to walk into a room and you had never met her, you would feel perfectly comfortable giving her a hug, and she would reciprocate. But if a brunette Winter Romantic such as Elizabeth Taylor walked into the room, and you had never met her, you would stand back and never touch her unless you were invited to do so.

A Romantic is a mature Ingenue. We all have a touch of the Romantic but it may not shine through until middle age.

A Gamin is a miniature, small-scale Natural. We have all known 80-year-old Gamins — wiry, active and independent. The Gamin is carefree and fast moving. She is the type who spends a thousand dollars for a week at a fat farm to be pampered and catered to, only to find that she'd really rather sweat it off on her own, running around the track.

The Ingenue possesses a deep, hidden source of femininity. After 16 years of age you are no longer a true Ingenue, but throughout your life you will have times when you need to reach deep down and pull up some of the intriguing, child-like, dependent qualities of this personality type. That is the feminine mystique.

This analysis is done in fun, but our observations are based on more than 20 years' experience in close association with thousands of women. Still, it is important to remember that each of you is unique, and each has her own amusing quirks and endearing qualities.

Yang Personality Analysis

	DRAMATIC	NATURAL	GAMIN
Body Type and Figure	Mature, Tall, Slender, Angular, Model Type. She can wear high-fashion.	Average to tall in height. Strong, sturdy body, broad shoulders. Athletic appearing. Wholesome outdoor type.	Small to medium height. Well-coordinated, miniature natural. May be slender, but never fragile looking. Sturdy, but never large in build.
Facial Features	Prominent, sharply-defined features. Definite coloring, usually Winter season.	Broad or long face, square jaw. Tanned, freckled. Natural appearing. Little make-up. Friendly, smiling eyes.	Small, rounded cheeks and chin or a square jawline. Turned-up nose, open, friendly happy face. Natural look, tanned or freckled. Mischievous sparkle in eyes.
Hair Style	Very plain, severe. Extreme high fashion.	Windblown, casual, short, unset, never fussy.	Short or long, straight or curly. Natural, windblown, casual styles. Wispy curls close to face.
Walk and Gestures	Poised, purposeful slow movements, firm and deliberate. Glides, with weight on heels.	Natural, casual, relaxed, energetic. Walks with a long, free-swinging stride. Stands with hands on hips.	Quick, skipping, free swinging walk. Sometimes awkward, but natural looking. Talks with hands, quick movements.
Behavior	Sophisticated, self-assured dignified, reserved, quiet.	Friendly, frank, open. Talks with hands. Suffers from "foot-in-mouth." Voice is strong, clear, of lower pitch, always friendly.	Alert, perky, bubbly, natural. Young at heart, friendly. Casual manner, tomboy, impatient. Outspoken.
Prototypes	Cher Bono, Lauren Bacall, Barbra Streisand, Shari Belafonte, Iman.	Carol Burnett, Shirley MacLaine, Julie Andrews Ethel Kennedy, Brooke Shields, Farrah Fawcett, Cheryl Tiegs, Christie Brinkley.	Sandy Duncan, Karen Valentine, Bonnie Franklin Sally Field, Mary Martin

Yin Personality Analysis

	CLASSIC	ROMANTIC	INGENUE
Body Type and Figure	Average height and body type. Balanced figure. Mature.	Average to short. Mature body, rounded feminine figure, full bust, rounded hips. May have a weight problem. large in build.	The most Yin type. Small-boned, dainty, feminine, often delicate looking. Gentle, rounded figure. Miniature Romantic.
Facial Features	Regular features. Medium to light coloring. Rarely of sharp contrast, often Summer season.	Soft rounded features. Large eyes. Flirtatious, natural feminine beauty. Rich coloring in any season. Stays young.	Rounded cheeks and chin. Dimpled, coy, demure. Fine boned. Delicate coloring. Large, innocent eyes.
Hair Style	Simple, neat, plain, but not severe. Soft controlled style.	Long, softly curled, feminine styles. Short feather cut. Soft bounce, never straight or stringy. Loose strands or ringlets.	Softly curled when long or short. Feather cut, soft bounce. Loose strands
Walk and Gestures	Poised, controlled, refined, lady-like.	Graceful, relaxed. Walks with a slow sway and feminine wiggle. May flutter when excited.	Graceful, dancing, light, airy. Reflects moods.
Behavior	Gracious, queenly, well-mannered, calm, conventional. Appears serene and contented. Pleasing, well-modulated, soft voice.	Charmingly feminine, softly sophisticated, flirtatious. Soft feminine voice.	Animated, shy, pouty. May appear naive, artless, and childlike. Appears young. Exact opposite of Dramatic. After 16, not a true Ingenue. Should have matured!
Prototypes	Grace Kelly, Dina Merrill, Pat Nixon, Nancy Reagan, Candice Bergen, Linda Evans, Catherine Deneuve, Margaret Thatcher, Queen Elizabeth.	Elizabeth Taylor, Gabor sisters, Jaclyn Smith, Ann-Margaret, Marie Osmond, Lynda Carter, Sophia Loren, Brooke Shields, Joan Collins, Victoria Principal.	Debbie Reynolds, Sandra Dee, Carol Lynley, Helen Hayes, Goldie Hawn, Charlene Tilton, Sally Struthers Bernadette Peters.

Your Total Image

Fabric, texture, clothing design, accessories and colors all have Yin and Yang qualities. Balance the blend of Yin and Yang in your choice of clothing with the blend of Yin and Yang in your personality. Each personality type has its own charm. The Yang quality gives opportunity for smartness, sophistication and high fashion. The Yin quality emphasizes beauty, charm and femininity. Youth is always a Yin quality. Maturity is a Yang quality.

Most people are a composite of two or even three types. It is important to harmonize the different qualities. This may be done by choosing costumes which avoid extremes in design of any one type, with emphasis on the more pleasing aspects of the individual's personal facial expression, coloring and figure. Emphasize whatever facet of your personality you may wish to enhance with any particular outfit, i.e., a Classic suit worn with a Natural tailored blouse for the office and a Romantic ruffled blouse for evening.

Instead of wishing you were different, learn to make the most of what you are.

DRAMATIC — She wears high fashion. The Dramatic woman can wear the simple, plain, tailored clothing for day and the extreme, exotic, costume look for evening. Fabrics are more often plain than patterned. If pattern is used, it is bold in color or value contrast, abstract or geometrical in form, and widely spaced. Textures may vary from firm weaves that tailor or drape well, such as crepe, broadcloth, gabardine and worsted, to soft jersey. Use lustrous fabrics for formal wear, such as satin, heavy brocade and lamé. Accessories vary from the bold, plain and large to the elaborate, ornate and lavish — long, heavy strands of beads or high chokers, large brooches, long hoops or chandelier earrings. Extreme, high fashion is designed for the Dramatic.

NATURAL — She is a casual, relaxed person and her casualness must always be suggested by the design of her clothing, even in afternoon or formal wear. Elegant sportswear is the Natural woman's best look. The straight silhouette is becoming. Plaids, checks, abstract, geometric or all-over prints look good on her. Uneven or rough textures like tweed, shantung, rough linen, raw silk or handknitted textures, and plain-surfaced fabric such as jersey, plain knits or gabardine are most attractive. Formal wear should be very simple in line, featuring beautiful fabric. Jewelry should be plain, chunky and natural looking, using plain metals, colored stones, Indian jewelry and large chains. The Natural uses restraint in clothing design and accessories, but not in quality.

CLASSIC — She is refined and ladylike. The Classic woman's clothing is essentially simple and dignified, fashionable, but never faddish or severe. The silhouette is basically straight, with fullness introduced in soft pleats or folds, never with a crisp bouffant look. Soft lines are most becoming. Plain fabrics are usually preferred, but soft florals, cascades and watercolor effects are good. Muted plaids, checks and polka dots are suitable. Medium- to lightweight fabrics such as fine silks, wool crepe, jersey, cashmere, fine cotton or wool broadcloth and other fine woolens are most becoming on the Classic woman. Dull-surfaced fabrics are preferred to those with high luster: chiffon, peau de soie or silk shantung are preferred to satin. Accessories are best kept simple. Jewelry should be modest, inconspicuous, smart and average size. Pearls are flattering. The Classic is the epitome of elegance at all times.

ROMANTIC — She wears soft, flowing dresses and lightly tailored suits with silky blouses, scarves and soft sweaters. Medium- to lightweight fabrics such as fine silk, crepe, jersey, plain knits, fine cotton, soft woolens and cashmere look best on the Romantic woman. For her evening out she wears velvet, lace, chiffon or peau de soie. Fur and feathers are especially becoming. For day wear she uses soft blended florals, polka dots, dotted Swiss, eyelet, embroidery, soft plaids and checks. Jewelry is dainty in detail but lavish in effect, curved of line and genuine. She likes to wear many pieces of jewelry and can get away with it if they are carefully coordinated. The Romantic is the epitome of femininity and sex appeal. Because she loves rich, pretty things, she must avoid the temptation to overdress.

GAMIN — Casual, snappy, chic is her theme. She can wear faddish accessories if scaled to her size. The Gamin's formal attire has an understated elegance. She is the typical skirt-and-sweater girl. The Gamin can wear small-scaled details, but she should avoid frills. Rick-rack is more her type. Scaled checks, plaids, stripes or stylized florals and small, abstract geometric prints look good on the Gamin. Crisp cotton, gingham, pique, linen, corduroy, soft tweeds and woolens, velveteen, silks, jersey, knits and novelty sheers are becoming fabrics. Jewelry should be kept to a minimum: lightweight chains, simple rings, pins. The Gamin should keep her clothing simple and wear interesting, quality accessories scaled to her size.

INGENUE — Because of her small build and youthful look, the Ingenue is able to wear the completely frilly frock of tucks, ruffles and lace or simple clothes in feminine fabrics. For day wear she uses lightweight soft woolens, cashmere, angora, fine silk and cotton, lightweight linen, jersey, knits, smooth voile or gauze. She likes small checks, blended plaids or stripes, polka dots and soft blended florals. For a dressier look she wears chiffon, organza, dotted Swiss, eyelet, fine silk, jersey and open crocheted-type knits. The Ingenue should avoid severe lines and too heavy or harsh fabrics. Soft textures and light hues suit her best. Accessories should be small, dainty and not extreme in style: small pearls, rhinestones for formal wear, or floral ceramic jewelry for daytime. Ribbons and bows are typical. As the Ingenue matures she should keep her clothing feminine but avoid a too young, "cutesie" look.

Each personality is unique in itself but the blending of Yin and Yang characteristics produce an infinite variety of women. Appreciate yourself for what you are and learn to express the different facets of your own personality in your choice of clothing, accessories, hair style and makeup.

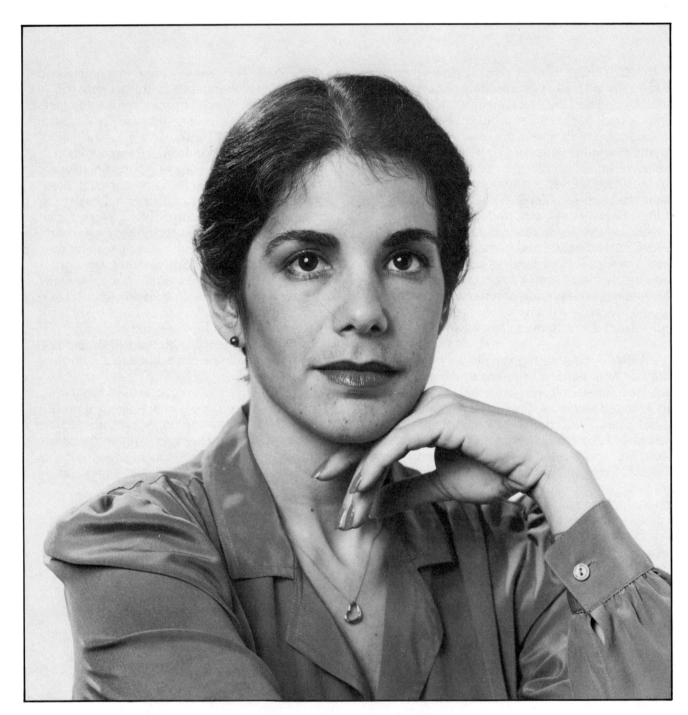

Tall and angular with definite coloring and facial features, Jennifer has a sophisticated high-fashion look.

Dramatic

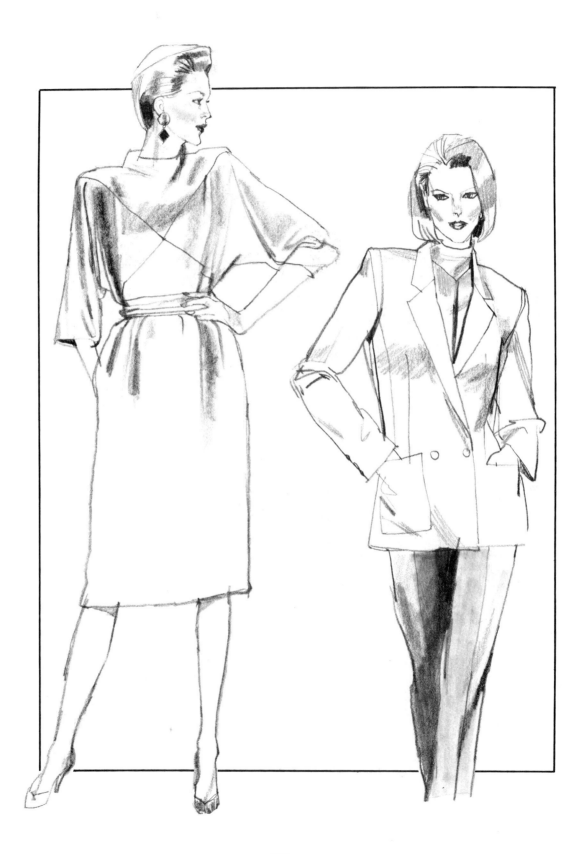

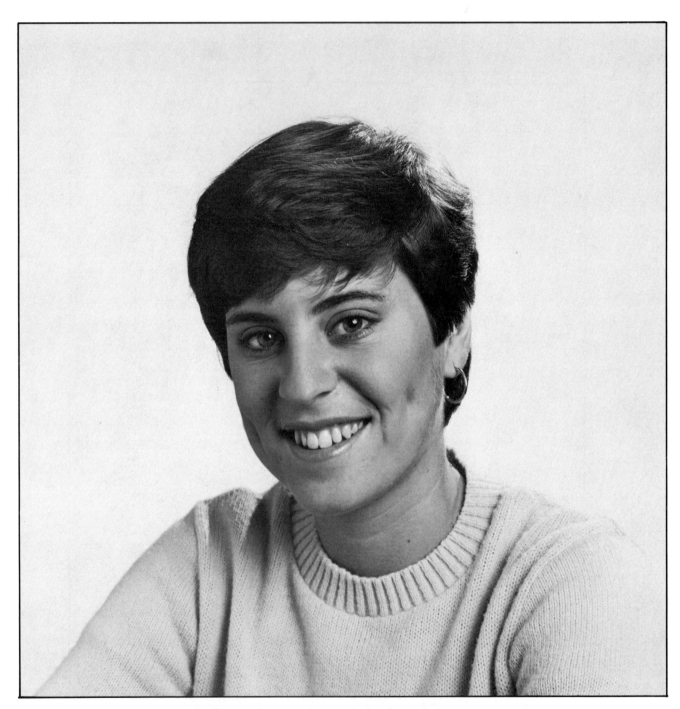

Cindy has a tall, sturdy body with broad shoulders. Her open, friendly smile and wholesome, outdoor look is typical of the Natural woman.

Natural

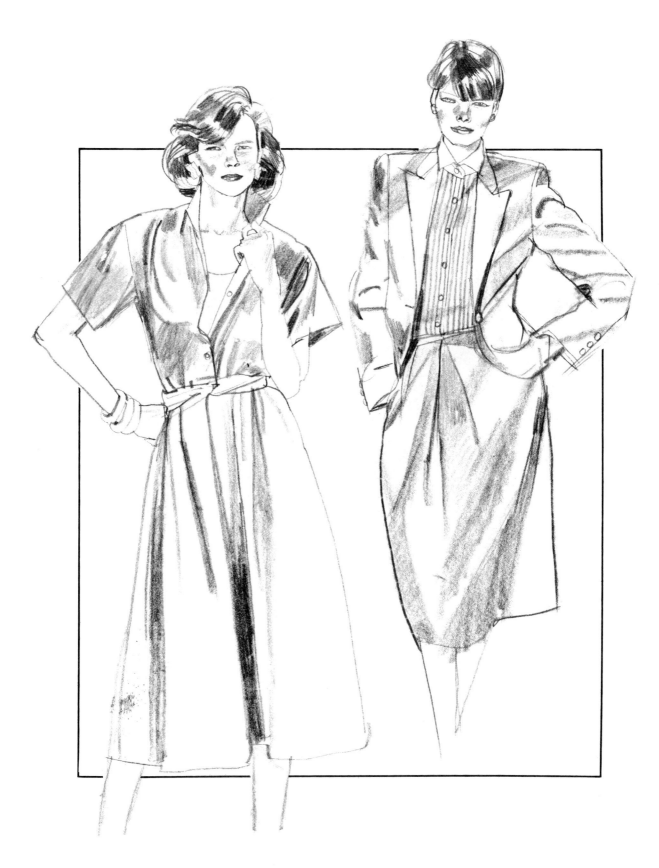

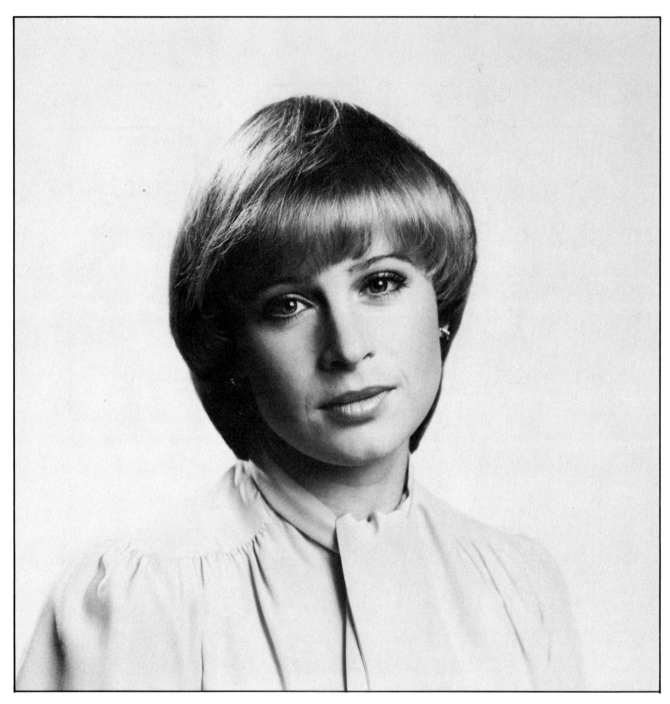

Poise, serenity and self-control typify the Classic woman. Anya has an air of gracious self-confidence.

Classic

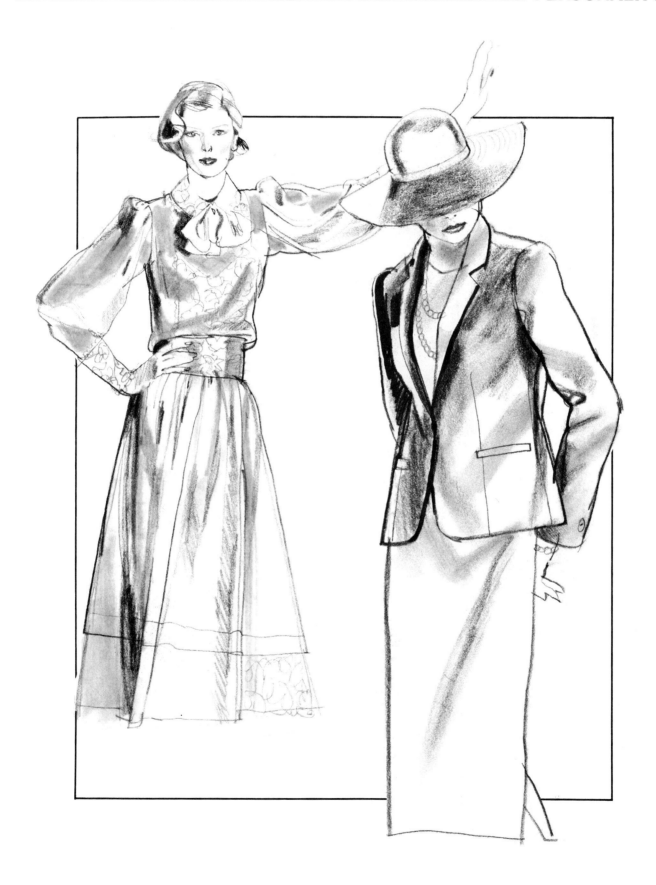

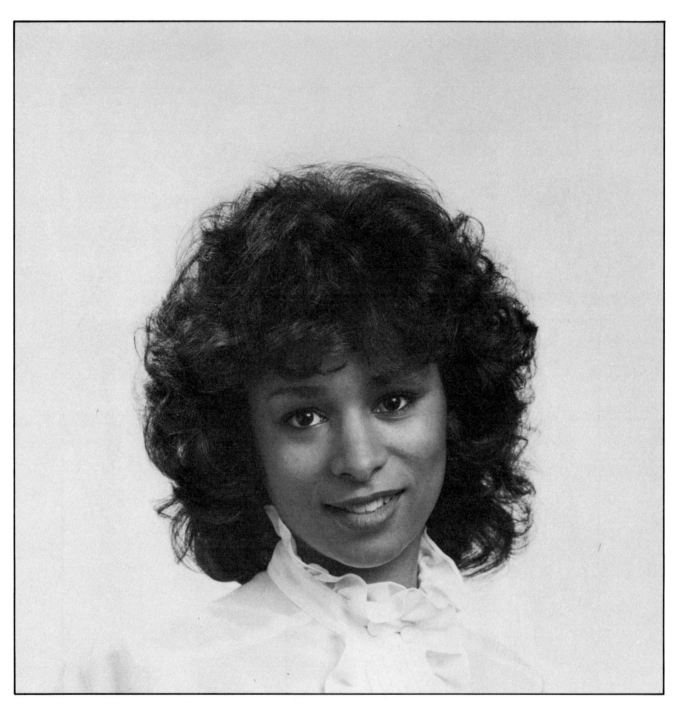

Charmingly feminine and flirtatious, Sharon has the large eyes and softly-rounded features of a Romantic.

Romantic

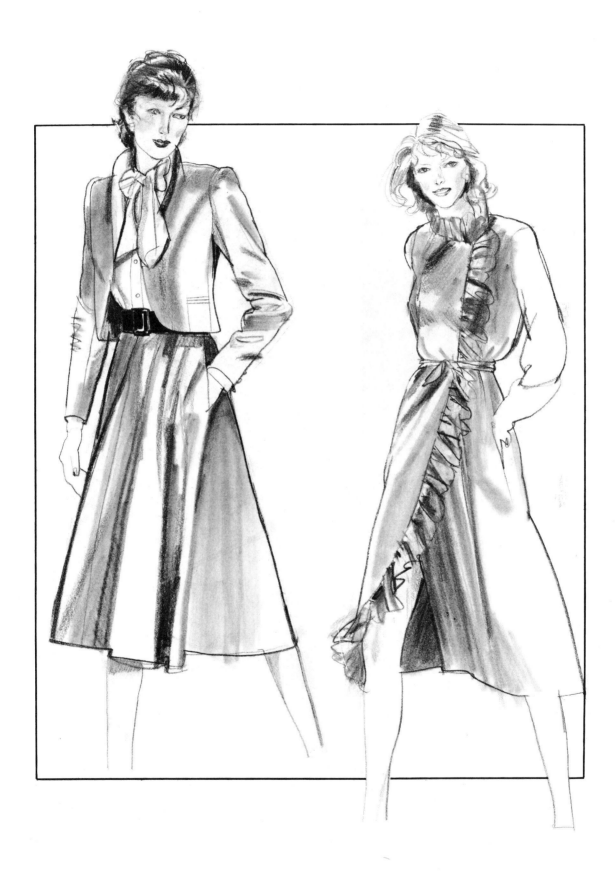

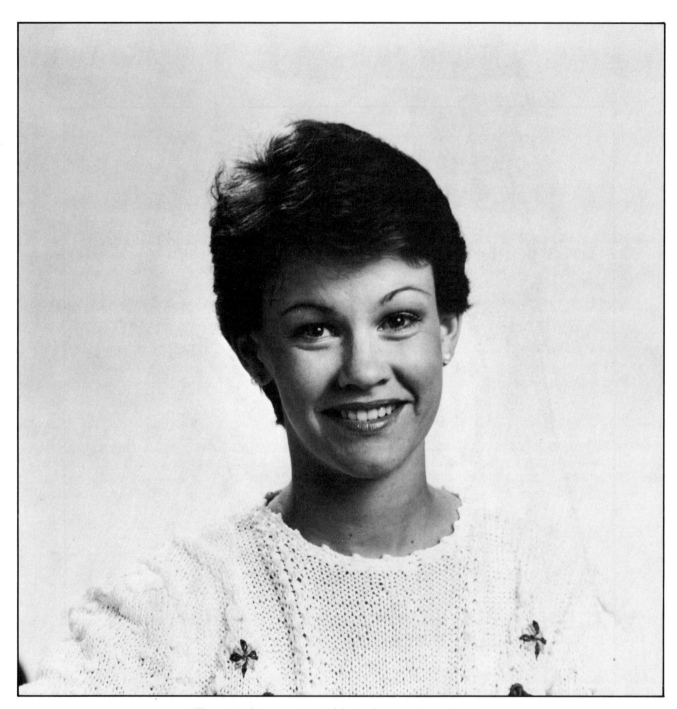

The mischievous twinkle in her eyes and her friendly, happy face identify Cindi as a Gamin. She is petite, but capable and perky.

Gamin

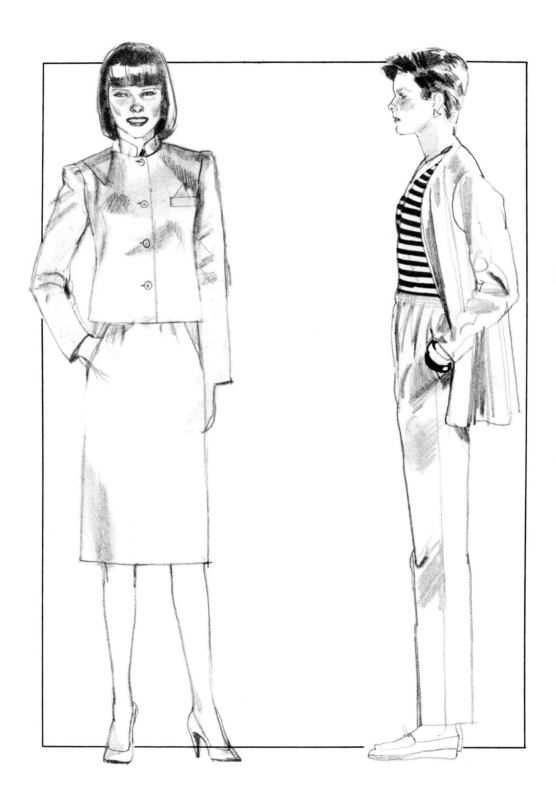

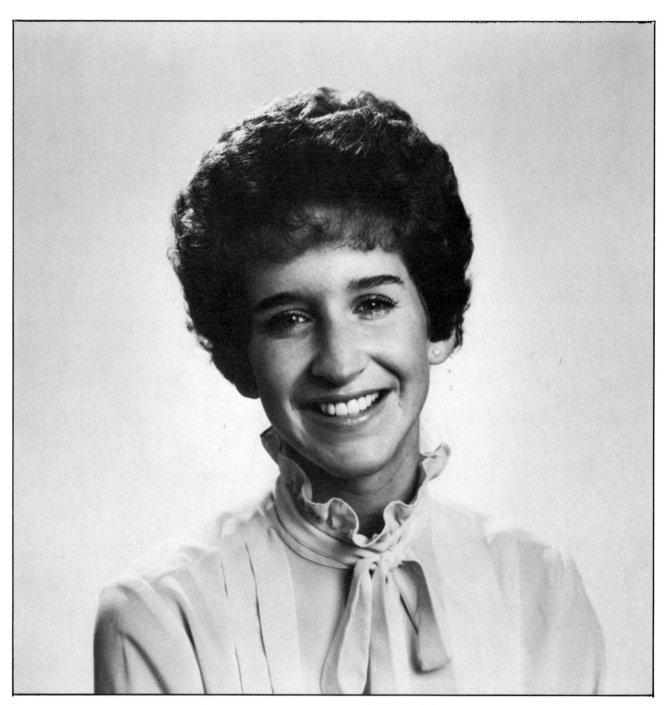

*Small-boned, feminine and delicate looking,
Tricia is graceful and animated. She looks
younger than her years, a miniature Romantic.*

Ingenue

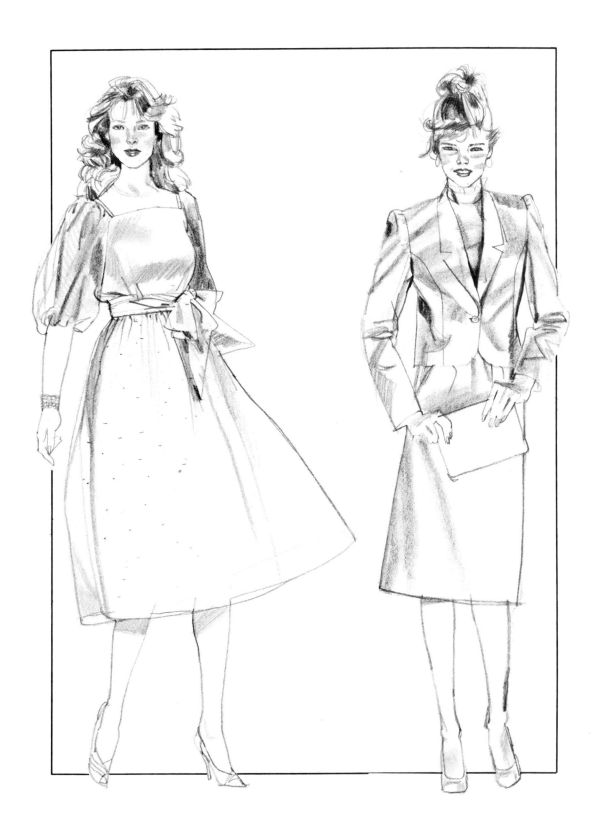

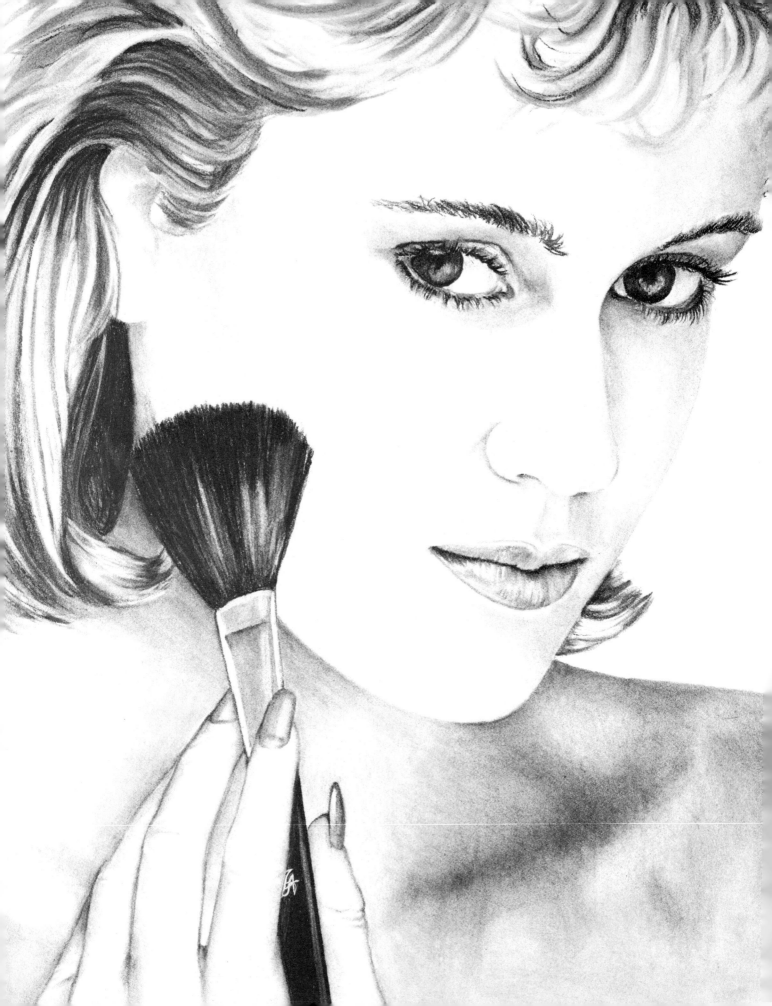

CHAPTER SIX

Skin Care And Makeup

BEAUTY IS ALSO SKIN DEEP

*A woman will look at 40
the way she deserves to look.*

There is no mystery and no magic about skin care. Skin care has primarily to do with comfort, protection and retention of a youthful look. As far as purity of product is concerned, you can use any brand you wish, purchased anywhere from the dime store to the highest priced cosmetic counter. In a skin care product you are looking for something with an agreeable texture, a pleasing fragrance, a pH balance and easy usability. Price does not determine quality. Buy whatever makes you feel precious, pretty and well cared for.

Skin, hair and nails are normally slightly acidic with a pH factor between 5 and 6. This "acid mantle" protects against bacteria and pollution. Any substance used on the skin which is either very alkaline or acidic will strip the skin of its protective covering. We feel it is important to use products which will maintain, rather than disturb, the pH balance of your skin and hair. Read the labels carefully on whatever skin care product you buy.

Skin care products are the most overrated, overadvertised and overpriced commodities in the world. We hope to bring some type of organization to the multitude of products offered by this multi-million-dollar industry.

We have heard so many divergent opinions about skin care that we are forced to conclude that no one has all the answers. It has long been our opinion that an excellent stress-free career would be dermatology. Dermatologists' patients rarely die of their skin disorders; they rarely recover from them either.

The skin is the largest organ of the body, covering about 18 square feet. It is controlled by heredity, diet during your lifetime, environment, the atmosphere, physical activity, your age, weight, amount of sleep and your general health. Your basic skin structure never really changes much. You just have to learn what works best for you. Get to know your own skin. It talks to you if you will listen.

Skin Composition

Skin is basically composed of three layers.

1. *Epidermis* is the outer layer, the part we see. This layer is continually shedding and will look flaky if the dead cells are not removed regularly. The epidermis has a protective film, called the "acid mantle," which counteracts bacterial infections and is most affected by cleansing products and cosmetics.

2. *Dermis* is the elastic second layer. The dermis is made up entirely of living cells, blood vessels, oil glands, sweat glands, hair follicles and nerve endings. The openings in the dermis are called pores. The sebaceous glands produce sebum, the lubricant which keeps the skin moist and soft, and constantly replenishes it. Sebum is slightly acidic and helps to preserve the acid mantle.

3. *Subdermis* is the third layer. This layer contains the fatty cushion cells. Blood vessels are most numerous here, and both sweat glands and

hair follicles originate in this layer. The sweat glands secrete perspiration, which flows out of the pores, carrying with it certain dissolved body wastes which have been stored in the subdermis. Wrinkles originate in this layer with the aging of the cushion cells. By the time a wrinkle appears on the surface of the skin, the damage has already been done.

Enemies Of Your Skin

The adversaries over which you have some control are excessive sun, alcohol, tobacco and crash diets.

Sunburn is self-inflicted skin damage. Everyone knows how to avoid it: either expose yourself gradually over a period of time to develop a suntan which acts as protection against a burn, or use sun lotions to protect your skin. A little sun gives good coloring and is healthful, but overtanning is aging, drying and conducive to skin cancer. As far as beauty is concerned, there is a point beyond which a tan is neither pretty nor feminine.

Alcohol causes capillary damage. It is high in calories and can be very drying to the skin. Alcohol and beauty do not mix, even in small amounts.

Tobacco makes the skin more sallow, yellows the teeth, dries the skin and contributes to wrinkling. There is a correlation between beauty and sweet breath. A smoker can never qualify.

A *crash diet* is any diet which does not include all basic nutrients. Lack of nutritional balance can produce sagging tissues, premature wrinkles and pale, lifeless color.

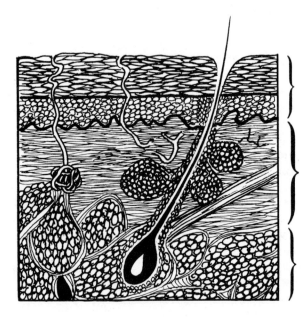

Epidermis: Outer layer, continually shedding

Dermis: 2nd layer, glands, blood vessels, hair follicles, nerve endings.

Subdermis: Fatty cushion cells

Basic Health Rules:

1. Get proper nutrition, especially plenty of fresh fruits and vegetables.

2. Get adequate rest. Try to avoid nervous tension.

3. Drink plenty of water (pop, coffee and tea do not count). Water is needed to hydrate the tissues and flush away toxic materials.

4. Maintain regular elimination. Roughage and bulk will help.

5. Develop a regular exercise plan. Run, walk, ride a bike, swim, do aerobic exercises. Exercise helps to relieve tension, tone muscles, firm skin and brighten skin tone.

6. Have a yearly check-up with your physician.

Skin Types:

1. *Normal* — This is the ideal skin. It is smooth and fresh, fine-textured, free of blemishes and neither dry or oily.

2. *Dry* — This skin appears thin and flaky. It feels tight and taut after washing. There is a tendency for whiteheads to develop. Dry, scaly patches on the face may prevent rouge or powder from going on smoothly. Dry skin is wrinkle-prone.

3. *Oily* — Oily skin is shiny and greasy, causing makeup to cake. It is usually coarse-textured, often accompanied by blackheads and large pores particularly around the hairline, nose and chin. You do not get rid of oily skin — you merely learn to control it.

4. *Combination* — This is the most common type of skin. This skin type will be oily around the nose, forehead and chin while the cheeks, temples and throat stay dry. Women over 25 are often in this category.

5. *Problem* — Problem skin is subject to skin disturbances such as acne. It can have an oversupply of oil, producing large pores, blackheads and blemishes. Problem skin is common among teenagers and becoming more frequent in adults.

6. *Sensitive* — Sensitive skin appears thin, sometimes pale. It has a tendency to flush easily and is most subject to allergies and broken capillaries. This skin type cannot be handled harshly or overstimulated. Sensitive skin is found in any skin type: oily, dry or normal.

Caring For Your Skin

Despite the dizzying array offered by the industry, skin care products fall basically into three categories: cleansing, toning and moisturizing.

CLEANSING — The first principle of good skin care is cleansing. A cleansing product removes makeup, skin secretions and dirt. Cleansing also stimulates circulation and keeps the skin looking healthy and alive. Cleansing should always be followed by toning and conditioning.

Never go to bed without cleansing your skin. For dry to normal skin, cleanse thoroughly at night; then in the morning you need only to sponge your skin with a damp cloth or wipe it off with a cotton pad dampened with your toner. Oily skin might benefit from cleansing two or three times a day. Go at your cleansing gently so as not to overstimulate. Many cleansing products are highly alkaline, which disturbs the acid mantle.

Cleansing Cream — Dry, normal or sensitive skin might use cream which is removed with a soft tissue or cloth. These products are too greasy for oily skin.

Cleansing Lotion — Cleansing lotion is most widely used by today's woman. It is a combination of oil and detergent and is removed with water. Preferred by the soap-and-water set, it does a thorough job. Lotion can be used by any type of skin.

Complexion Soap — Usually preferred for oily skin, complexion soap can be drying for other types. Soap is always alkaline and strips the acid mantle. If you like soap, use a facial bar.

Scrubs — Scrubs are massage-type stimulators. The grains help remove the dry, flaky epidermis and loosen embedded dirt and oil. If dry skin appears flaky and dull, it will be helped by weekly use of a scrub. Oily skins could use a scrub more often. Scrubs have a refining influence on large pores.

Masks — You can stimulate circulation by using a mask. It temporarily helps to remove the tiny network of wrinkles and fatigue lines, toning and tightening the skin. A mask can be a beautifier for a special evening out.

TONING — A toner acts as a mild stimulant which brings the blood closer to the surface to nourish and moisturize the skin. It also helps to tighten the pores and restore the acid mantle of pH balance. Always follow cleansing with a toner to remove any traces of oil. Do not use anything too strong on the face. A toner should just tingle for a minute, not burn or hurt.

Freshener-Toner — The freshener-toner is milder with less or no alcohol. It is better for normal to dry skin.

Astringent — A slightly stronger toner, the astringent usually contains more alcohol. It is preferred by normal to oily skin types.

MOISTURIZING — Most skin would benefit from some type of moisturizer to help protect it from soil, smog, dust, wind and sun. Moisturizers do not add oil to the skin, they only help skin retain its own natural oils and moisture which keep the skin soft and supple. Always apply very sparingly. Moisturizers help makeup go on smoothly and prevent it from clogging the pores. You may need to change the texture of your moisturizer from summer to winter due to climatic differences.

Lotion — Lotion is of a lighter texture, used for normal to dry skin in humid summer months. Oily skin should use exceptionally light-textured moisture lotions which utilize humectants rather than oil. A humectant is a moisture-retaining or moisture-giving substance that can be absorbed by the skin.

Creams — Dry, normal, sensitive or combination skins may be helped by rich, light-textured creams which blend moisturizers and emollients that actually add oil and hold moisture throughout the day. Emollients are used as night creams for dry skin but are too rich for oily skin.

Extras For The Woman Who Likes To Pamper Herself

Eye oils and throat creams are rich blends of emollients and vitamins A, D or E. These are often very expensive but you may feel they are worth it. Hope springs eternal.

All of us grow older, but we wish the side effects of aging, especially the visible ones, did not have to be a part of the process. Cosmetics and skin care products can make us feel better and look younger, but cosmetic chemists and medical people have yet to cure the effects of aging. Your goal should be a lifelong commitment to a healthful regimen and the regular application of whatever products you find most effective and pleasing.

Good diet and vigorous exercise, will improve your health and the appearance of your skin. Skin care products should also make your skin feel better and look more cared for. You should realize, however that the product by itself does little. Skin care products encourage your skin through stimulation, sedation or nourishment, to take care of itself. After you have done all you can do to help your skin you are ready to add radiance with makeup coordinated to your season.

Putting Your Best Face Forward

In our opinion the best-looking women have a natural look. One does not achieve a natural look by running around with a naked face. Some women need a bucket of makeup to look "natural." Properly applied makeup should emphasize your best facial features and be keyed to your total personality.

Cosmetic companies would have us change our whole technique each season to keep up with the current fashion-magazine face. This may be good for their corporate image but won't do much for yours. You need to recognize that they are more interested in peddling products than making the most of you.

Most cosmetics come out of the same pots. Two or three large cosmetic laboratories produce most of the makeup in the United States, except for the real biggies like Revlon, Max Factor, Avon, etc., which produce their own. This is a highly specialized field. These fine laboratories have the equipment, skilled personnel and stringent quality control required to produce lipstick, rouges, pressed powders, eye shadows, etc. All cosmetics sold in the United States meet the standards set by the Food and Drug Administration and are considered pure. However, purity has nothing to do with allergic reaction. Allergies are caused by certain ingredients, such as fragrances, lanolin or PABA, to which your skin objects. The basic ingredients of cosmetics are practically the same, as is the cost. The color, texture and fragrance will vary, however. The retail cost of makeup will vary depending on the packaging and the quality of the advertising.

Makeup fashions do change, but the changes are subtle — from lighter to darker lipstick, from heavy eyeliner to none at all, from false eyelashes to heavy mascara. Fashions also vary in the placement of rouge and the technique of applying shadow. All of these will change and at times seem extreme, but over the years we have noted that the pendulum always swings back to the pretty, feminine, natural-looking face.

Good makeup techniques are fairly standard. Your own particular method should be determined by your facial structure and coloring. You might modify as years go by, but you should not make radical changes once you learn the most becoming method for you.

Makeup is an art and takes time, patience, practice and good lighting. Makeup should be a supplement, not a concealment.

Experimenting can be expensive. That drawerful of wrong colors can represent quite an investment.

In buying cosmetics you are buying color and texture. The color we hope to help you with. But the texture is a matter of skin type and personal preference, whether you like a cream rouge as opposed to a blush, for example. The amount of makeup you wear should be determined by your activities, your age and your personality type. A young girl may need only a lip gloss and some blush. The older you get, the more makeup you need — but the color must be softened. If you can't see clearly what you are doing, buy a triple mirror.

At the Fashion Academy we see a lot more women wearing too little makeup than we ever see wearing too much. And we have heard every excuse in the book as to why they don't wear it. The actual fact of the matter is that most women who wear too little makeup are either too lazy or are in a quandary over how or what to put on.

We are going to lay some ground rules on makeup use, but unless you experiment intelligently and try these techniques, you will never find your new image — and discovering your best look should be your goal.

Foundation

Foundation base is used primarily to enhance the texture of your skin, to blend in complexion flaws, freckles, blemishes and color variations. Foundation should add a flattering tone to your skin, increasing color in the case of sallowness. When you buy a foundation and later find you need a pound of rouge to look healthy, you can be sure that your foundation is too flat and does not have enough color in it.

There are different textures of foundations: cream, liquid and cake. Your skin type determines which texture you should use. Oily skin prefers a water-base liquid or cake. A normal to dry skin may prefer liquid or cream.

The skin must be clean before applying a foundation. Foundation must be used sparingly and will go on more smoothly if applied over your moisturizer while the moisturizer is still dewy damp.

COLOR — Foundation comes in two basic undertones: rose, which is cool, and yellow, which is warm. Be aware when buying a foundation that many salesclerks cannot distinguish between warm and cool undertones and have not been properly trained to choose a foundation for you.

First, you must determine whether the foundation you are considering is cool or warm. You do this by comparing one with another. Second, to find the right shade, you apply a tiny drop to your chin line and gently pat and blend. Never apply foundation on the neck. Your neck is usually one shade darker than your face. Ideally the foundation will create a blend between the neck and face. You should not be able to see where the makeup ends.

Too light a color gives a mask-like effect and the fine facial hairs become noticeable.

The foundation which most closely matches your skin tone can be worn nine months of the year. For the summer months when you are tan, change to a shade or two darker in the same undertone. Sometimes it is hard to find the in-between shade. Instead, you can mix a little of your darker foundation with the regular shade if they are the same brand.

FACE POWDER — A translucent (no color)— powder is best. When properly applied, powder eliminates the shine, thus giving a matte-finish look. This is especially recommended for oily skin.

To apply: Dust loose powder lightly over face with a brush or a clean ball of cotton, lightly brushing off excess with a complexion brush.

Powder is applied over your foundation and cream rouge, but before powder rouge, eye makeup and lipstick.

SUGGESTED FOUNDATION COLORS:

Winter: (Rose tone)
Natural pink (fair skin)
Rose-beige
Deep rose-beige
Dark rose tan
Avoid: Yellow tones; they will look orange.

Summer: (Rose tone)
Natural pink (fair skin)
Rose-beige
Deep rose-beige
Avoid: A too-pink tone.

Spring: (Yellow tone)
Ivory (fair skin)
Peach
Warm beige
Deep peach (when tan)
Avoid: Dark suntans

Autumn (Yellow tone)
Ivory (fair skin)
Peach
Warm beige
Deep peach
Suntan (when tan)
Avoid: Drab warm beige; you will look sallow.

Rouge or Blush

Next to lipstick, rouge is the most effective cosmetic you can wear. It gives a glowing healthy look and emphasizes the good points of your bone structure. We place cream rouge after the foundation and before loose powder. Powder blush is applied after loose powder. We place it on the height of the cheekbone and blend it out to the hairline. Smile and blend the color on the fullness of your cheek. This technique looks more natural, as if the sun put the color there. It also lifts the face and makes the eyes sparkle.

Several textures of rouge are available. Cream rouge is good on normal to dry skin. Oily skin may respond better to brush-on powder blushers.

Because the cheek is the driest part of the face, rouge will go on easier if it is applied over a little moisturizer. Use sparingly and blend to perfection. Too much rouge can look worse than none at all.

Rouge: No closer to nose than center of eye. No lower than nose.

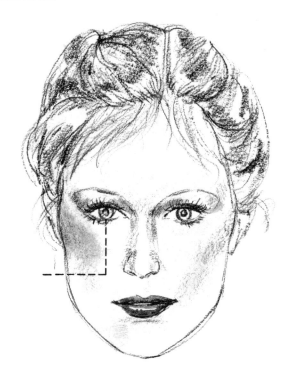

SUGGESTED ROUGE COLORS:

Winter: (Rose tones)
Rose
Wine
Red (true)
Avoid: Peach, rust or brown shades;
your cheek will look dirty.

Summer: (Rose tones)
Pink
Rose
Wine
Avoid: Yellow tones — peach, bronze, etc.

Spring: (Yellow tones)
Peach
Coral
Red (clear)
Avoid: Deep peach or browns

Autumn: (Yellow tones)
Tawny peach
Brick
Red (clear)
Avoid: Brown shades.

Lipstick

Lipstick adds color to your face and makes the teeth appear white. Master the use of a brush to perfect a balanced lip line. You could survive with just two lipsticks, but most women have many.

There is no way to predetermine what color a lipstick is going to be without trying it on your lips. Due to the acidity of your system, the color can change. The purple undertone in the lips of some Winters and Summers causes lipstick to seem too dark. Winters often need a more vivid lip color with their bright or basic colors. If the lipstick seems too bright, some Winters have found it helpful to dab a touch of cool lip toner over or under the color to tone it down. The alternative is to choose a more dusty shade of Winter's medium to dark colors.

Fair, blonde Summers can wear the lighter, dusty pinks, but the darker Summers need a deeper shade of their rose-pinks.

Springs have the least trouble finding lipstick colors. They just need a good peach and coral.

Autumns have trouble with their lipsticks turning pink. A warm lip toner used over or under the lipstick may be helpful. Autumns have the hardest time finding good lip colors. They will have the best luck mixing a light and a dark shade together. Brown lipstick is not good. Brown is not a natural lip color. Autumns should stay in the terra cotta and rust tones.

Lip glosses are for young girls. Mature women need more color. Women with gray hair should avoid lipstick that is too dark, too bright or frosted. Frosted lipstick can be worn by Romantic personalities. The earth tones of Autumn do not adapt well to frosted lipstick, except for evening wear.

Nail Polish

Manicured nails are imperative for a well-groomed look. Don't let your nails get too long; claws are grotesque.

It is best to keep your nail polish in a soft, light to medium dusty shade. Avoid the darks and brights except for a special costume look. Soft-colored nail polish improves the looks of all hands. Bright, glaring, frosted nail polish is not a tasteful daytime look. Frosted lip and nail color is better for evening use and on Romantic personalities.

SUGGESTED LIPSTICK AND NAIL COLORS:

Winter: (Rose tones)
Rose-pinks and blue-reds
Wines and burgundies
Reds (true)
Cool lip toner
Avoid: Warm-tone burgundy and browns.

Summer: (Rose tones)
Pink and rose
Mauve and plum
Burgundy and wines
Avoid: Too-harsh blue-pinks.

Spring: (Yellow tones)
Peach and honey
Coral and salmon
Poppy red and watermelon
Avoid: Rusts and browns.

Autumn: (Yellow tones)
Peach and apricot
Ginger
Rusts
Brick reds
Warm lip toner
Avoid: Browns and rose-tone rusts.

Eyes

Your eyes are the focal point of your face. This is where most women fail with their makeup — they either do nothing or overdo. Harmonize eyebrow pencil, eyeliner and mascara with your hair color.

EYEBROWS — The brow should start directly over the inner end of the eye. The thickest part of the brow should be kept in this area and it should taper up toward the middle. The highest point should be in line with the outer edge of the iris, then the brow should curve out and down slightly to the end of the eye. Never tweeze above the brow. Tweeze only on the forehead between the brows and under the brows. Fill in the brow if needed with feathery, short strokes of a pencil, brushed through, to intermingle with the natural hairs. *Never make a solid, hard line.* The color must always be as close to the color of the natural hair as possible. Test by putting an eyebrow pencil mark on the forehead to see how the natural oils affect the color.

SUGGESTED COLORS FOR EYEBROW PENCIL:
Winter:
Charcoal gray
Black-brown
Soft black
Dark brown
Taupe
Gray (with gray hair)
Avoid: Browns with red in them.

Summer:
Taupe
Black-brown
Charcoal gray
Gray
Silver-beige (blondes)
Avoid: Browns with red in them.

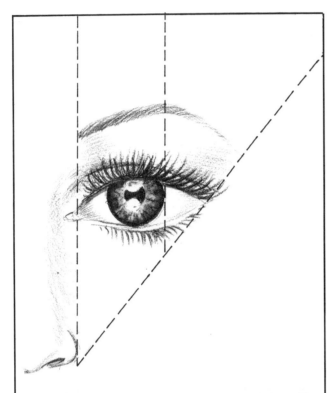

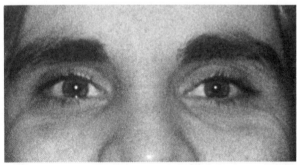

Untweezed Eyebrows

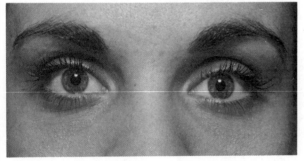

Same Eyebrows Tweezed

Spring:
   Light brown
   Taupe
   Medium brown
   Silver-beige (blondes)
   Gray (with gray hair)

Autumn:
   Light brown
   Medium brown
   Dark brown
   Taupe
   Gray (with gray hair)

EYELINER — Eyeliner gives depth to the eye and makes the lashes seem more lavish. Everyone does not need eyeliner. If your lashes are light in color, however, you will benefit. Start your liner at the inner corner of the eyelash, using a very fine line drawn as close to the lashes as possible. The outer corner of the eye is the outer limit! Never apply liner below the eye and never use black — it is too harsh. When liner is applied on the bottom lid, it makes the eye appear smaller and look as if your mascara is smudged. Use a Q-tip™ to correct goofs and to thin out a thick line. Eyeliner is applied before shadow because the blending of the shadow softens the eyeliner.

SUGGESTED COLORS FOR EYELINER:

Winter:
   Black-brown
   Charcoal gray (with blue or gray eyes
   or gray hair)
   Avoid: Browns with red in them.

Summer:
   Brown
   Black-brown
   Gray
   Avoid: Browns with red in them.

Spring:
    Brown
    Gray (with gray hair and gray-blue eyes)

Autumn:
    Brown
    Black-brown

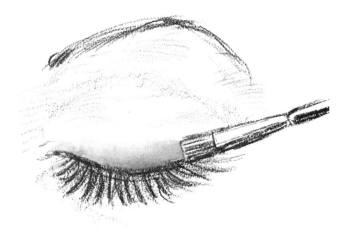

EYE SHADOW — The purpose of eye shadow is to enhance the eyes. It can intensify the color and size, but must be used with care. Eye shadow should harmonize with the eye color, not the costume.

Eye shadow comes in powders, creams and crayons. We prefer powders because they are easiest to blend and work with. You must use a good sable brush. A Q-tip™ can be used to help in blending or removal of any excess that may have fallen below the eye on the cheek area.

Cream and crayon eye shadow works most successfully on dry, crepey eyelids. Crayons are fun to use for accenting.

The secret to using an eye shadow is in the blending.

For a special effect, a touch of eye crayon may be applied below the outer, lower lash, extending inward only ¼-inch (.5 cm) to ½-inch (1 cm).

We work with three areas: the lid, the crease and the flesh on the orbital bone (brow bone).

If you use color, it should be placed on the lid close to the lash. The color used should blend with your eye color, preferably a shade to bring to life the lightest color in the eye. Sometimes a neutral is placed over the color to soften it. If your shadow color is more noticeable than the color of your eye, you blew it! A color on the eye is not always necessary. Neutrals often work best. (See charts on pages 8-25 for suggested eyeshadow techniques.)

The way you apply shadow on the rest of the eye is determined by whether your eye is *deep-set, prominent* or *standard*. Different techniques may be used. To bring out a sunken area, for instance, we use a light neutral; to make a protruding area recede, we use a darker neutral.

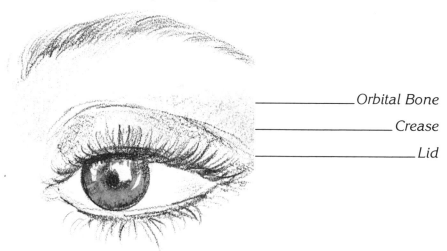

_____*Orbital Bone*

_____*Crease*

_____*Lid*

MASCARA — Most eyes benefit from the use of mascara. It darkens the lashes and makes them appear longer and thicker. Those who wear contact lenses will be more comfortable if they apply eyeliner to the base of the lash and mascara only to the tips. This helps to keep mascara off the lenses. Also apply mascara to the bottom lashes.

SUGGESTED COLORS FOR MASCARA:

Winter:
   Black-brown
   Black
   Charcoal gray (with gray hair)
   Avoid: Browns with red in them.

Summer:
   Brown
   Black-brown
   Charcoal gray (with gray hair)
   Soft black (apply sparingly)
   Avoid: Browns with red in them.

Spring:
   Brown
   Black-brown

Autumn:
   Brown
   Black-brown

FALSE EYELASHES — False eyelashes add glamour. The individual clusters which you can learn to apply yourself are the most comfortable and practical if you wear lashes all the time. If you manage to find a good glue, they stay on for weeks. Strip lashes are fun for a special occasion. False eyelashes are a terrific lift for a mature face. We recommend short lashes because even medium lengths are too long . Winters should use black lashes. Summers, Springs and Autumns use brown-colored lashes.

The colors and techniques suggested in this chapter are basic. Experiment with others, but don't fall into the fad trap. Individuality is the key to successful makeup. You have to find your own unique style. You do this first by experiment, then by practice.

While developing your own style of makeup, you need to consider your crowning glory — your hair style.

Prominent Eyes

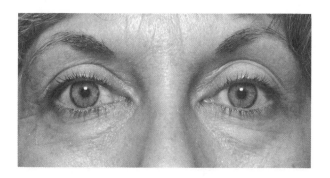

The way you apply shadow on the rest of the eye is determined by whether your eye is **deep-set**, prominent or **standard**. *Different techniques may be used. To bring out a sunken area, for instance, we use a light neutral; to make a protruding area recede, we use a darker neutral.*

Standard Eyes

Standard Eyes (fleshy bone and eyelid)

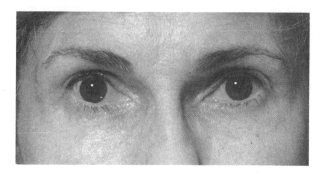

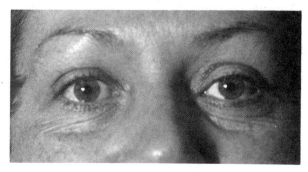

Deep-set Eyes

Deep-set Eyes (fleshy bone, no lid)

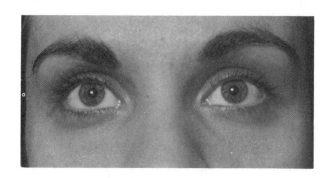

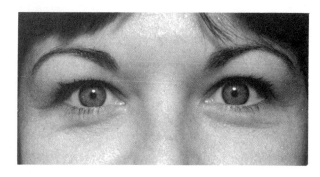

Winter Eyeshadow Techniques (L=lid; C=crease; B=bone)

Eye Color	Deep Set Eyes	Prominent Eyes	Standard Eyes
Blue or Gray-blue	L—Soft gray, misty blue C—Bisque, beige, pink beige B—Beige, gray, navy	L—Gray, smoky blue, navy C—Gray, smoky blue, navy B—Gray, smoky blue, navy	L—Gray, smoky blue, navy C—Gray, beige, smoky blue, navy B—Gray, smoky blue, navy
Green or Gray-green	L—Soft gray, sea green C—Bisque, beige, pink beige B—Gray, bisque, beige	L—Gray, gray green, smoky turquoise C—Gray, smoky turquoise B—Gray, smoky turquoise	L—Gray, gray green, smoky turquoise C—Gray, beige, smoky turquoise B—Gray, smoky turquoise
Blue-green (aqua)	L—Beige, gray, smoky turquoise C—Bisque, beige, pink beige B—Gray, bisque, beige	L—Gray, smoky turquoise C—Gray, smoky turquoise B—Gray, smoky turquoise	L—Gray, smoky turquoise C—Beige, gray, smoky turquoise B—Gray, smoky turquoise
Hazel (brown-blue-green)	L—Gray, smoky turquoise C—Bisque, beige, white, pink beige B—Gray, bisque, beige	L—Gray, smoky turquoise C—Gray, smoky turquoise B—Gray, smoky turquoise	L—Gray, smoky turquoise C—Beige, gray, smoky turquoise B—Gray, smoky turquoise
Lt. Brown (yellow-green)	L—Beige, gray, smoky turquoise C—Bisque, beige, white, pink beige B—Beige, gray, smoky turquoise	L—Gray, smoky turquoise C—Gray, smoky turquoise B—Gray, smoky turquoise	L—Gray, smoky turquoise C—Beige, gray, smoky turquoise B—Gray, smoky turquoise
Brown	L—Beige, gray, navy, smoky mauve, smoky turquoise C—Bisque, beige, white, pink beige B—Beige, gray, navy, smoky mauve, smoky, turquoise	L—Gray, navy, smoky turquoise, smoky mauve C—Gray, navy, smoky turquoise, smoky mauve B—Gray, navy, smoky turquoise, smoky mauve	L—Gray, navy, smoky turquoise, smoky mauve C—Beige, gray, navy, smoky turquoise, smoky mauve B—Gray, navy, smoky turquoise, smoky mauve

These are suggested colors, but you should experiment for the proper effect for your own eyes. Gray is a basic neutral for Winters. We never use brown, it makes your eyes look tired. Silver may be used in place of gray for evening and a soft white or bisque to highlight under brow. Beware of bright pinks and plums unless Pink Beige or Smoky Plum, or you will look as if you have been crying.

Summer Eyeshadow Techniques (L=lid; C=crease; B=bone)

Eye Color	Deep Set Eyes	Prominent Eyes	Standard Eyes
Blue or Gray-blue	L—Soft gray, soft blue, misty blue C—Bisque, beige B—Gray, navy	L—Gray, soft blue, smoky blue, navy C—Gray, smoky blue, navy B—Gray, smoky blue, navy	L—Gray, soft blue, smoky blue, navy C—Beige, gray, smoky blue, navy B—Gray, smoky blue, navy
Green or Gray-green	L—Gray, aqua, sea green, smoky turquoise C—Bisque, beige B—Gray, smoky turquoise	L—Gray, aqua, sea green, smoky turquoise C—Gray, smoky turquoise B—Gray, smoky turquoise	L—Gray, aqua, sea green, smoky turquoise C—Beige, gray, smoky turquoise B—Gray, smoky turquoise
Aquamarine	L—Gray, aqua, smoky turquoise C—Bisque, beige B—Gray, smoky turquoise	L—Gray, aqua, smoky turquoise C—Gray, smoky turquoise B—Gray, smoky turquoise	L—Gray, aqua, smoky turquoise C—Beige, gray, smoky turquoise B—Gray, smoky turquoise
Hazel (Chameleon)	L—Gray, aqua, smoky turquoise C—Bisque, beige B—Gray, taupe, smoky turquoise	L—Gray, aqua, smoky turquoise C—Gray, smoky turquoise B—Gray, taupe, smoky turquoise	L—Gray, aqua, smoky turquoise C—Beige, gray, smoky turquoise B—Gray, taupe, smoky turquoise
Brown (soft)	L—Gray, taupe, smoky mauve C—Bisque, beige B—Gray, taupe, smoky mauve	L—Gray, taupe, smoky mauve, navy C—Gray, taupe, smoky mauve, navy B—Gray, taupe, smoky mauve	L—Gray, taupe, smoky mauve, navy C—Beige, gray, taupe, smoky mauve, navy B—Gray, taupe, smoky mauve, navy

Gray is a basic neutral for Summers. Taupe is seldom used, and only on hazel or brown eyes. Use gray over blue or green shadow to soften it. Never use yellow greens. Experiment but keep it soft. Highlight under the brow with bisque. Summers have too much pink in the eyelid to wear pink or plum shadows. You will look as if you have been crying.

Spring Eyeshadow Techniques (L=lid; C=crease; B=bone)

Eye Color	Deep Set Eyes	Prominent Eyes	Standard Eyes
Blue or Blue-gray	L—Beige, taupe, gray, smoky blue, soft blue C—Bisque, beige B—Beige, brown, gray, smoky blue	L—Taupe, gray, soft blue, smoky blue C—Taupe, gray B—Taupe, gray, smoky blue	L—Taupe, gray, smoky blue, soft blue C—Beige, taupe, gray B—Taupe, gray, smoky blue
Green (yellow)	L—Beige, brown, taupe, sage green C—Bisque, beige B—Beige, brown, taupe	L—Taupe, brown, sage green C—Taupe, brown B—Taupe, brown	L—Taupe, brown, sage green C—Beige, taupe, brown B—Taupe, brown
Blue-green (aqua)	L—Beige, taupe, smoky turquoise, aqua, gray C—Bisque, beige B—Beige, brown, taupe, gray, smoky turquoise	L—Taupe, brown, gray, aqua, smoky turquoise C—Taupe, brown, gray, smoky turquoise B—Taupe, brown, gray, smoky turquoise	L—Taupe, brown, gray, aqua, smoky turquoise C—Beige, taupe, brown, gray, smoky turquoise B—Taupe, brown, gray, smoky turquoise
Hazel	L—Beige, brown, taupe, gray smoky turquoise C—Bisque, beige B—Beige, brown, taupe, gray, smoky turquoise	L—Taupe, brown, smoky turquoise C—Taupe, brown, smoky turquoise B—Taupe, brown, smoky turquoise	L—Taupe, brown, smoky turquoise C—Beige, taupe, brown, smoky turquoise B—Taupe, brown, smoky turquoise
Lt. Brown (golden)	L—Beige, brown, taupe C—Bisque, beige B—Beige, brown, taupe	L—Brown, taupe C—Brown, taupe B—Brown, taupe	L—Brown, taupe C—Beige, brown, taupe B—Brown, taupe

Springs have a delicate coloring and in keeping with their natural look their makeup should be applied sparingly and blended well. Browns applied too heavy will make your eyes look tired. Bisque is used to highlight under the brow. Gray shadow can be used for blue eyes or gray hair. Avoid yellows, coppers or rusts, which make the eyes look sallow and tired.

Autumn Eyeshadow Techniques (L=lid; C=crease; B=bone)

Eye Color	Deep Set Eyes	Prominent Eyes	Standard Eyes
Lt. Brown (amber)	L—Beige, taupe, brown C—Bisque, beige B—Beige, taupe, brown	L—Taupe, brown C—Bisque, beige, taupe, brown B—Taupe, brown	L—Taupe, brown C—Bisque, beige, taupe, brown B—Taupe, brown
Brown	L—Brown, beige, olive brown C—Bisque, beige B—Brown, beige	L—Brown, olive brown C—Brown, olive brown B—Brown, olive brown	L—Brown, olive brown C—Beige, brown, olive brown B—Brown, olive brown
Green (golden)	L—Taupe, brown, moss green, olive green C—Bisque, beige B—Beige, taupe, brown	L—Taupe, brown, moss green, olive brown C—Brown, taupe B—Taupe, brown, olive brown	L—Taupe, brown, moss green C—Beige, taupe, brown, olive brown B—Taupe, brown, olive brown
Hazel	L—Beige, taupe, brown, smoky turquoise C—Bisque, beige B—Beige, taupe, brown, smoky turquoise	L—Taupe, brown, smoky turquoise C—Taupe, brown, smoky turquoise B—Taupe, brown, smoky turquoise	L—Taupe, brown, smoky turquoise C—Beige, taupe, brown, smoky turquoise B—Taupe, brown, smoky turquoise
Teal Blue (turquoise)	L—Beige, taupe, brown, smoky turquoise C—Bisque, beige B—Beige, taupe, brown, smoky turquoise	L—Taupe, brown, smoky turquoise C—Taupe, brown, beige B—taupe, brown, smoky turquoise	L—Taupe, brown, smoky turquoise C—Beige, taupe, brown B—Taupe, brown, smoky turquoise

Gray or taupe may replace brown shadow when hair is gray. Browns applied too heavy will make the eyes look tired. Reddish browns such as copper, ginger, rust, or yellow, etc. will make the eyes appear red and look like you have been crying. Apply brown over green to tone it down. Bisque is used to highlight under brow. No blue shadows for Autumn except Smoky Turquoise. Experiment but be objective and blend. Makeup on Autumns should look natural.

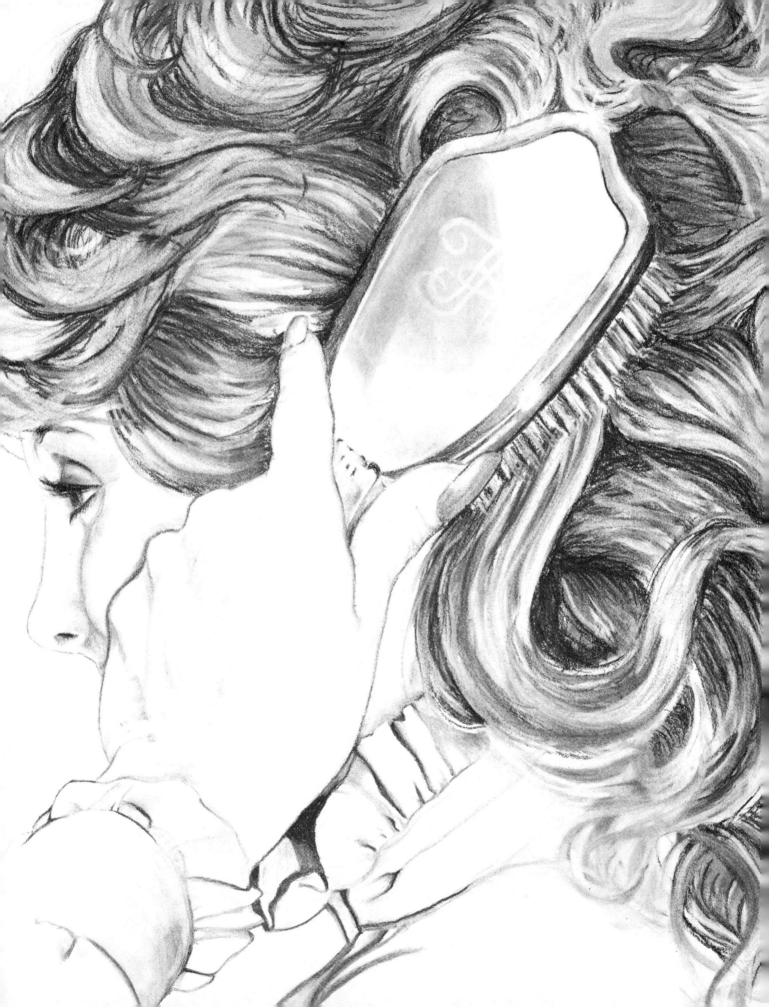

CHAPTER SEVEN

Hair

YOUR CROWNING GLORY

Sue had traveled from another state to have her hair styled. She had been waiting for weeks and had a specific cut in mind. She told us exactly where she wanted each hair to fall. Then we went to the stylist with her.

"Well, Sue, what are you going to have this time?" he asked. She sat demurely in his chair (an attitude not in keeping with her decisive Winter personality) and answered, "Oh, anything you think would be nice."

Our first impulse was to scold Sue until we realized how common her behavior was. A woman is either intimidated by hairdressers or assumes they are clairvoyant, able to discern her wants by reading her mind.

The biggest problem between you and your hairdresser (a more critical relationship than with your gynecologist) is one of communication and rapport!

Hair is the single most important factor in looking good. Your hair should be your crowning glory. If your hair looks good, you feel good.

Finding a good stylist and then giving him or her the chance to become acquainted with your hair, your personality and your lifestyle takes time and some sleuthing. Watch for others with hair texture similar to yours whose styles you admire. Ask for a recommendation. Then give the stylist a chance if the initial vibes are good. You need one who will listen to you and who is sensitive to your needs. He or she needs the opportunity to work with your hair, learn how you live and how much skill you have in handling your own hair.

The foundation of a style is a good cut. It takes three months to correct a poor cut, especially if the hair is worn short.

A hair style is determined by the shape of your face, the length of your neck, the slope of your shoulder, the texture of your hair, your body proportion and height, your age, your personality and your lifestyle.

In discussing hairstyling we usually use the term "trim," because women develop instant trauma if we say "cut."

Length

Hair grows from one-half (1 cm) to three-fourths (2 cm) of an inch per month, and somewhat faster in warm weather. Summer is a good time to grow a new hair style.

Women with square shoulders or short necks can achieve better balance if they keep their hair off the shoulders. The hair in back should be tapered in a V effect rather than rounded. Gray hair is best worn medium to short, cut regularly and always well-groomed.

Short — Under four inches at the crown, two inches at sides and back, and an inch at the bottom, tapering to nothing at the neckline. Short hair needs frequent trimming, every three to four weeks.

Medium Short — Four to five inches at the crown, tapered to about ear-tip length at the sides. It should be trimmed every four to six weeks.

Medium — Five to seven inches all over the head, two inches at the nape of the neck, falling to a length just below the chin line. Medium hair needs trimming every four to six weeks.

Medium Long — An inch or two above the shoulders. It should be trimmed every five or six weeks.

Long — Shoulder length or longer. Long hair can be done up; any length that can be pinned up can be considered long hair. Long hair should be trimmed every six to eight weeks.

Hair Style

The ideal shape of face is an oval. You should strive for a hair style that will create a well-balanced, oval illusion. If you have regular facial features and the right personality, you may get away with extreme hair styles.

OVAL — Oval-shaped faces with regular features may wear most styles, even drawn back in sleek lines. Oval faces with irregular features or mature faces will benefit from styles that are softened around the face.

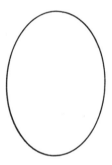

OBLONG OR RECTANGLE — Your goal is to give width and minimize length. Keep hair full at the sides, using minimum height at the top. A side part is best unless bangs are worn to reduce the length of the face. Center-parted, long-hanging, shoulder-length hair is not becoming unless shaped shorter and fuller at the sides of the face.

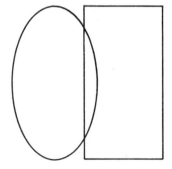

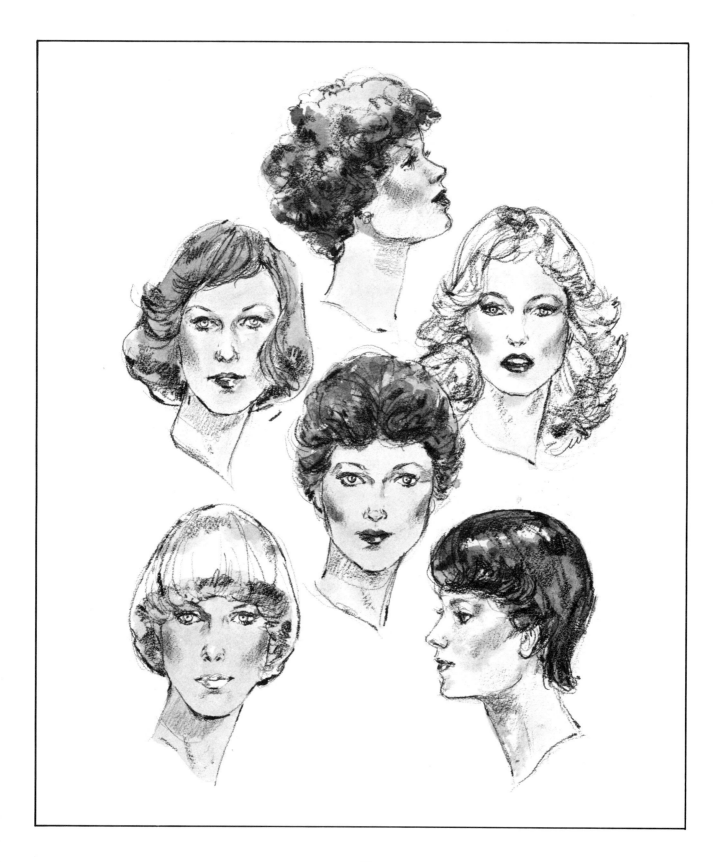

ROUND — The round face requires the illusion of length or height to diminish its moon shape. Wear a center part only if hair covers the sides of the forehead and sides of the face. A side part should be a diagonal line toward the crown. Height is needed at the crown, keeping fullness above the ears. Dip hair onto cheeks to minimize width of face. Pulling the hair away from the face is too severe unless you are a Dramatic personality.

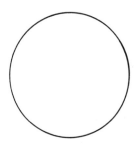

SQUARE — You need added height to achieve a more oval illusion. Asymmetrical lines are best. Keep fullness away from the jaw line. Layered or broken lines soften the face. Do not expose the entire forehead hairline or wear an extremely low side part.

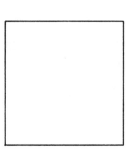

PEAR OR TRIANGLE — For a pear-shaped face, softly irregular curled or wispy bangs with a flare toward each side may be worn. Keep hair close to the cheek line, partly covering the ears, to soften a wide jaw.

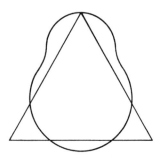

HEART OR INVERTED TRIANGLE — Your goal is to achieve symmetry between a broad forehead and a narrow chin. A soft, feminine

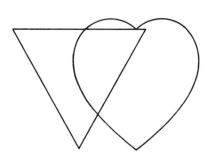

coiffure is preferable. Avoid low side parts, severely tailored lines or a top-heavy look. Hair is best worn swept high across the forehead, lying fairly close at the top of the head. This is the face shape which best wears the long, loose, full, tapered hair that falls to the shoulder, adding width to the jawline.

DIAMOND — You need to broaden the forehead and jaw areas to balance with the cheek. Symmetrical lines are good. Swirled or feathered bangs across the forehead are effective to provide width, keeping hair full at temples but close at cheekline. You may wear your hair short or long. Keep fullness around your jawline if hair is worn long.

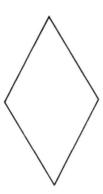

Keep your style up to date. Adapt your basic shape to the current trends. Never wear your hair too short, because it gives a mannish look. After 25 the hair should be off the shoulders, at least in front because long hair accentuates any lines in the face. In fact, after 25 everything should go up but the hemline. A center part is the hardest to wear because it accentuates any irregularity in the facial features. An asymmetrical line is easier to wear.

Hair Color

We have never met a woman whose natural hair color did not go with her skin and eyes. Mother Nature did an excellent job, but we too often decide that we know better. When our grandmothers got bored or needed a lift, they went out and bought a new hat. Modern women color their hair instead — often with drastic results. Don't misunderstand, we are not opposed to artificially-colored hair; we just want you to stay close to your own natural color. It is imperative that you stay with the same undertone or you will create a disharmony with your skin and eyes.

Naturally gray hair, when dyed too dark or too bright, will look harsh against the skin which has prepared itself for gray hair. Mature women who dye their hair must choose a shade or two lighter than their original color or it can be aging and look unnatural.

In choosing a color for your hair, recognize that regardless of the color shown on the dye charts, your hair will end up at least two shades darker. To achieve the most natural-appearing colored hair, you must use several colors of dye. For this reason, it may be cheaper in the long run to have your hair colored by a professional because you cannot keep the dye for your next job, but he or she can finish up a partially-used bottle within its time limit.

Regardless of what you may have heard, using henna to create shine or add color to your hair is a mistake unless you are an Autumn. Henna adds an artificial red-orange color to brunette Winters and Summers.

In your search for a hairdresser, recognize that all hair stylists are not necessarily skilled with color. Color is an art, and not all hairdressers are artists.

Highlighting The Hair

Frosting is done by putting a cap on your head, then pulling strands free with a crochet hook and bleaching them clear down to the roots. Frosting should be done very lightly, and only on natural blondes where their hair may have darkened slightly. Summers are the only ones who can wear frosted hair successfully. Dark brunettes should *never* frost their hair. It will age them 10 years. Frosting turns the hair of an Autumn drab gray and her skin cannot handle the changes.

Highlighting is another method of frosting done by taking small strands of hair, applying a lightener and wrapping them in plastic or foil. It takes longer but the results are prettier.

Painting is done while the hair is combed into its regular style. Colors or lighteners, or a combination of the two, are applied with a brush. The pressure applied and the timing determines the result. Some light Autumns look good with this method of highlighting.

Luminizing is a Clairol Corp. trade name. It is a mild treatment to lighten and brighten dull hair. Timing is critical. Luminizing looks good on Springs and Autumns. Summers beware — your hair will look brassy.

If all these methods of highlighting are performed by a skilled operator, the results are harmonious. If done by an unskilled person, however, the hair can look over-colored and cheap.

Frosting has a growout problem. The tendency is to refrost too often, giving the hair an overly-bleached look. Highlighting, painting and luminizing have the advantage of a less noticeable grow-out, and all of them need to be done less frequently than frosting.

Many times what your hair needs is conditioning with moisturizers and protein to restore its sheen, rather than highlighting. Of prime importance to beautiful hair is a healthy diet.

Too many women fool around with their hair color when they do not know what they are doing. If your hair is graying and you are not ready for it, obtain the help of a good beauty operator to find a color shade close to your natural hair color.

Winters and Summers should stay in the cool, ash tones. Springs and Autumns should stay in the warm, golden tones. Autumns can use red for highlights.

Baby-fine and straight hair is often dyed, hennaed or frosted, in the hope that it will get body. It would be safer and more successful if the hair were given a body wave.

You are getting it all together! You have discovered yourself from your season's colors to hair design. You are ready now to adapt them all to your lifestyle.

CHAPTER EIGHT

Discovering Lifestyle

CLOTHES FOR THE LIFE YOU LEAD

In order for you to develop personal style, every outfit you acquire must be right for you in terms of color, line, personality and lifestyle. A good wardrobe is built around your way of life, but lifestyles change from year to year. A change of employment, change of residence, your marital status, the growth of your children and your age all influence lifestyle and your clothing needs.

One of the notable gratifications in life is to be thought of by your peers as a well-dressed person. You will never gain that reputation by being the most casually-dressed woman at the activities you attend. People who are considered well dressed are always dressed one level better than everyone else — not two levels better, or they will hate you. The trick is to observe carefully what your associates wear, socially and professionally, and then take the trouble to improve your own choices so that you always look just a little bit better than they do. Of primary importance, of course, is wearing the colors that are right for you. The rest of the technique is more subtle and has to do with the clothes themselves.

First, improve on the type of garment you wear. For instance, when you go to a casual meeting, everyone else may be wearing pant separates; you wear a matching pant set. If they wear matching pant sets, you wear a pant suit. If they wear pant suits, you wear a skirt suit because a skirt always looks better than pants.

Second, improve the quality of the outfit. This is done with better fabric, better tailoring, better fit and perfect accessories. They wear polyester; you wear a natural fiber or a polyester that *looks* like a natural fiber. They carry plastic handbags; yours is genuine leather. They have lots of inexpensive clothes; you have a few excellent clothes.

It is not the *quantity* that makes your reputation, it is the *quality*.

Most of our students thought they understood their clothing needs. The results of the following exercise, however, came as a revelation to them as it will to you. To know what you need in the way of clothes and accessories, you need to know exactly where you go and what you do.

1. Keep a record for twenty-four hours a day. A well-dressed person is well dressed twenty-four hours a day. When we say well dressed, we do not necessarily mean "dressed up." We want you to be dressed in the best garment of its kind for the activity in which you are engaged. If you are scrubbing floors you should be dressed for floor scrubbing, but if you run out of wax and have to run to the store for more, you should change your clothes. Why? Because who do you meet at the store — everybody. And the worse you look, the more people you meet.

2. Keep your daily record for three weeks. This period should cover most of the different places you go. If daily activities in the same garments are repeated, record the outfit only once.

3. Repeat the exercise two or three times during the year to make yourself aware of how your needs change with the climate.

4. Repeat the exercise every three to five years to keep abreast of lifestyle changes.

5. Each day write down where you went and what you wore. Then do some fantasizing, and write down what you think would have been the best possible outfit you could have worn for that particular activity. For example: "Went to kitchen to cook breakfast. Wore faded old robe which should have been replaced years ago. Wish I owned a cheerful, colorful, washable, comfortable housecoat."

6. Also record any special needs for occasions such as an annual ball, a cruise, vacations, etc.

In three weeks your third column will show you where your wardrobe is failing to work for you. This list will be the basis of a Priority Shopping Plan that you should start acting upon now. List the important purchases you wish to make as you begin to build your wardrobe for your new image.

Now that you are aware of clothing requirements for your lifestyle, you need to clean out your closet and drawers and get organized.

Clear The Decks

Plan a whole day for this chore. Open your closet door and survey the accumulation of a lifetime: skirts you have had since college, dresses from before you gained or lost weight 10 years ago, shoes with pointed toes and needle heels. You are allowed to cry a little, but then get down to business. Most closets are jammed with things we never wear.

Start with the clothes. Take everything out and dump it on the bed. Vacuum the closet and attend to moths and silverfish. Sort your clothes into three piles according to the chart on page 141.

WARDROBE PLANNING FOR MY LIFESTYLE 24 Hours a Day for 3 Weeks 2 to 3 Times a Year Every 3 to 5 Years		
Where I Went	*What I Wore*	*What I Wish I Had Worn*

WEARABLES — *Everything that is ready to wear goes back in the closet.* Even though some garments may not be in your colors, put them back because no one can afford to discard good wearables. We have found that once our students find their best colors they never want to put the wrong ones on again. But put them back anyway. If the seams are intact, all the buttons are attached and the garments are clean, you may be able to put a scarf, blouse or sweater with that wrong black or brown slack or skirt. Use them up, wear them out until they can be replaced. There may not be many clothes left in your closet — how refreshing!

REPAIRABLES — A repairable is any item worth saving that is not immediately wearable. Pile repairables wherever you put things in need of attention — in your sewing room, in a spare closet, or in a pile to go to the drycleaner.

DISCARDS — Those things in your closet which you have not worn for a year, with the exception of a ball gown or other specialized garments, discard or donate to your favorite charity. Chances are you will never lose those extra pounds. If you are waiting for the style to be resurrected, forget it. The silhouette might return but something will be different — the fabric, the color, the emphasis of fit, the shoulder pads or the length. If you find blouses you have not worn, you either have too many blouses or not enough skirts and slacks to go with them.

Repeat the discard process with your shoes and bags, in your bureau drawer and your jewelry box. An exception to the discard rule is your jewelry. Anything good, bright and like new which you are not wearing, place in a plastic bag and store. It might return to fashion. Save those old girdles or Merry Widow bras for posterity or the rare occasion when you might feel the need for one.

It is a good idea to store shoes in the garage. Any that you have not retrieved after a year, give away.

ANALYSIS OF MY WARDROBE		
Wearables	*Discards*	*Repairables*

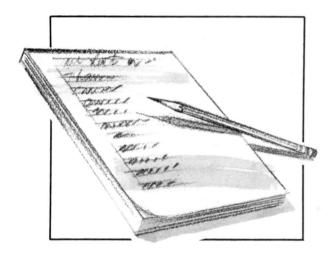

Make A List

From those few lonely clothes you have hanging, uncrushed, in your closet, cut a fabric sample out of the seam allowance or hem. If you made a garment or shortened it, you may be able to get a two-inch swatch. Then, on a large safety pin, collect these samples of your clothes. This is your wardrobe record to carry in your purse. It is imperative to carry these samples when shopping, to help match and coordinate new purchases, because twenty seconds after you turn your back on a color, you cannot remember its exact shade. Your safety pin is just that: a reminder.

This idea was born after Joyce, a student, lost her slacks while carrying her new pant suit through the mall, searching for a blouse. She was left with an orphaned jacket. Carrying clothes for matching is irksome and tiring.

List what you have and note any new purchases you want to add to make each garment more suitable — scarf, blouse, jewelry, etc. Add these items to your Priority Shopping Plan and you are on your way with a wardrobe plan for your *New Image.*

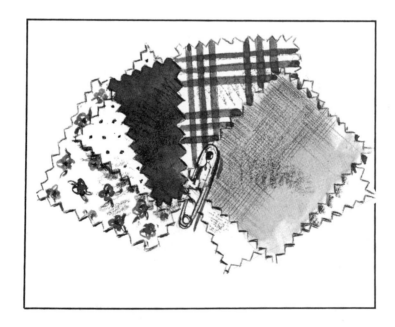

CHAPTER NINE

Wardrobe Planning

ORGANIZING AND COORDINATING YOUR WARDROBE

Using Colors In Planning Your Wardrobe

Color is exciting and can open up a whole new world for you. The key to successful buying and wardrobe planning lies in your choice of color. Never buy clothes or accessories unless the color of your new purchase is keyed to your wardrobe plan. Every color you wear must have a purpose, be related, and most of all, do something for *you*.

Plan your wardrobe around your neutrals. Neutral colors are whites, grays, black, navy, beiges and browns. They are basic and will go anyplace, any time. Each season has its own basic neutrals. Choose your neutrals to harmonize with your hair and eyes. Your basic shoes and bag should be in your neutrals. A costume of all neutral colors is most elegant if hair is well groomed, makeup properly applied and you are feeling well and have had adequate rest.

For wardrobe planning we also include the *basic colors* which are reds, blues and greens in medium to dark shades. They are not neutrals, but they will go most anyplace, any time. They are becoming because they add color to the face. Basic colors are good used for coats, suits, dresses, blouses, sweaters, etc.

Choose one or two neutrals around which you will plan your wardrobe, possibly varying with the time of year. This will simplify the choice of accessories and help to insure color unity. Keep your neutrals in mind when adding other colors to your wardrobe.

Use Of Neutrals And Basic Colors In Wardrobe Planning

BLACK — A particularly good choice for city wear or for dressy occasions, black is sophisticated, smart. Black is worn best by Winters. If you are not a Winter, and there is enough black in a garment to require black accessories, don't buy it.

BROWN — Brown's light to medium shades are essentially more casual, natural and informal. Brown becomes sophisticated and dressy when used in a very dark value. It is used in place of basic black for Autumns, who can wear most shades of warm brown. Springs wear only rich, warm, medium shades of brown. Summers wear rose-browns shading to burgundy. Winters wear no brown except a very dark brown which could be worn with black shoes.

NAVY — An excellent choice for any season of the year, Navy is much kinder than black and beautiful with gray hair or blue eyes. Navy adapts well to tailored classic costumes for both young and old and is good for sportswear. A clear, warm, royal navy replaces basic black for Springs. A gray-navy (French) is a good basic for Summers. A true navy suits Winters best. Autumns should wear teal blue instead.

GRAY — Becomingness varies greatly with the value and intensity of the gray. This is a very adaptable basic color, particularly for the basic coat, suit or dress. Gray takes on different qualities in relation to the colors used with it. It gives a conservative, classic look. This neutral can be most becoming, elegant and chic when a shade has been chosen to harmonize with gray or graying hair, or blue eyes. Choose the gray of your season: clear, warm grays (dove) for Springs; light to medium blue-grays for Summers; light to dark true grays or blue-grays for Winters; grayed browns (coffee) for Autumns.

BEIGE — Beige is similar to gray in its variable character, and it looks attractive on all seasons, depending on the value and intensity selected. It is often used for a basic, classic coat. Beige is usually most becoming to those with brown hair. Gray-beige is best for Winters, rose-beige for Summers and warm yellow-beige for Springs and Autumns.

WHITE — Any season can wear a true off-white; it is most versatile. Chalk-white for Winters is fresh and crisp-looking for spring and summertime, and very elegant for winter formal wear. Few other seasons can wear chalk-white successfully unless it is worn away from the face, mixed in prints or worn in the summertime when the wearer is tanned. Summers wear only a true off-white. Ivory or yellow-whites are better for Springs or Autumns.

RED — Red is almost as basic and easy to work with as a neutral. It proves most acceptable as a coat or accessory color to coordinate with the wardrobe. Bright orange-reds or true reds are best for casual wear. Blue-reds are a better choice for dressy wear. Wine, burgundy or plum are good choices as a basic color for Summers, maroon, crimson and true ruby red for Winters. Rust is a good basic for Autumns. Clear, warm red is a good accent for Springs.

BLUE — Everyone likes blue. It is a basic color, conservative and classic. True blues are best for Winters, gray-blues (cadet) for Summers, teal-blues for Autumns, clear blues for Springs. Hot, bright blues are not considered basic. They are worn for fun day wear or sophisticated evening wear in rich fabric. Lighter, softer blues give a more delicate, feminine look for summer day wear or an elegant look for evening. Aqua or medium turquoise is a good basic for summertime wear or in warmer climates.

YELLOW — Yellow is basic in the gold shades only for Autumns and Springs. Most people are rightfully afraid to wear yellow. It is one of the most difficult colors for Winters and Summers to wear. However, Autumns and Springs will find yellow one of their most becoming colors. Yellow is great for active sportswear and a good accent used with navy and brown on casual clothes.

GREEN — Warm, muted greens, from the lightest shades to the darkest olive, are some of Autumns best colors and are excellent used as a basic in her wardrobe. Clear, warm greens in light to medium shades are good for Springs. Summers can wear most shades of blue-greens. True green, like yellow, is a more difficult color for Winters to wear unless mixed with white, and then it is not a basic. Blue-greens are more becoming on Winters and are more elegant and dressy.

BRIGHT COLORS — These colors are more intense, medium to dark shades. They are used as bright accents with neutrals or mixed in prints. They are fun colors for active sportswear. If used solid in a large area, such as a dress, the fabric must be of good quality or it can look cheap. Bright jewel colors make very sophisticated evening wear when made of a rich fabric and simple design.

LIGHT COLORS — Pastels and ice tones are more feminine and delicate. They look good in lingerie, dressy blouses, scarves, summer wear and evening dresses with a fuller, more feminine design.

A Workable Wardrobe Plan

If you had absolutely nothing to wear and someone gave you money to put together a wardrobe, where would you start? Most women assume that they should start with a coat, suit or dress. This is not true. To plan a workable, infinitely expanding wardrobe, you must start with shoes and bags. Look up the color charts on pages 8-25. After determining from the charts which neutrals are yours, explore the stores to see which of your neutrals are being shown this season.

An ideal first choice would be a neutral from your palette which can be worn nine months of the year, one which is readily available on the market and one which will coordinate with your existing collection of clothes. There are times when the choice of neutral shoes and bag is limited, such as the five years during the '70s when there was little shown in chocolate brown and the winter of '80-'81 when there was no navy blue.

Give careful consideration to *availability* and *coordination* with what you already have, make your decision, and use discipline to stay with your plan until it is complete.

Refer to the chapter on accessories for variations in the styles of these shoes and bags which can be used for your basics according to your personality type and lifestyle.

This kind of a wardrobe can take from two to five years to develop, depending on how much time and money you have available. Don't get frustrated and don't get sidetracked. When you realize that your wardrobe is starting to come alive and work for you, it is exciting and worth all the effort.

BASIC NEUTRALS FOR SHOES AND BAGS

Winter
Black (essential)
Navy (essential)
Gray (optional)
Maroon (optional)
White (summer)
Gray Bone (summer)

Summer
Navy (essential)
Wine (essential)
Gray (optional)
Rose Brown (optional)
Rose Bone (summer)

Spring
Navy (essential)
Milk Chocolate (essential)
Camel (essential)
Warm Gray (optional)
Yellow Bone (summer)

Autumn
Dark Brown (essential)
Rust (essential)
Camel (essential)
Med. Brown (optional)
Olive (optional)
Yellow Bone (summer)

The difference between a summertime and wintertime wardrobe is a matter of texture, weight and color. The old rule states that summer starts with Easter and ends in September. In Florida, Hawaii and warm climates, however, summer goes on all year 'round.

A Basic Wardrobe Plan

A good wardrobe should contain at least one of each of the following items. Your lifestyle will dictate in which areas you need more. For example, every woman needs at least one skirt suit. A professional woman might need several, but the young homemaker and mother of small children needs only one suit with many casual coordinates.

Your first set of shoes and bags will all be the same color.

Your first set of shoes will consist of:

Your first set of bags will consist of:

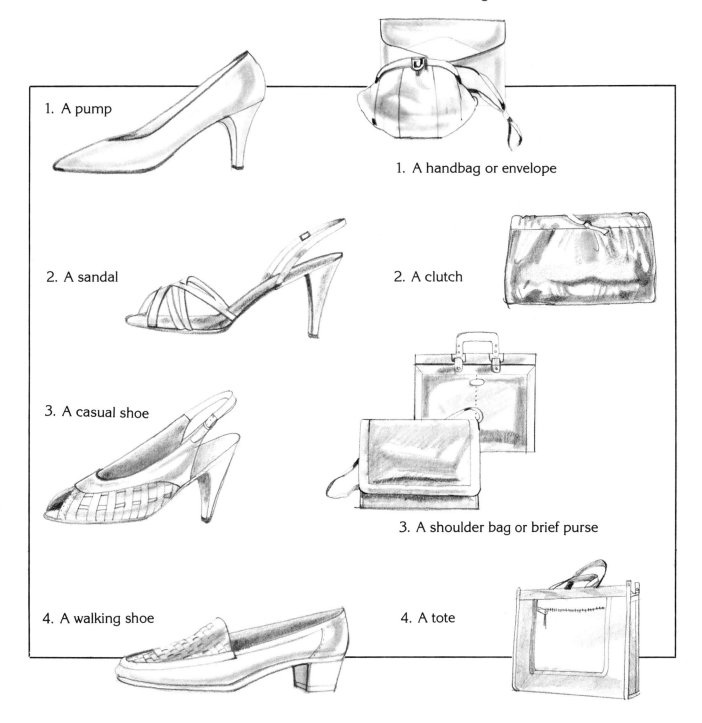

1. A pump

2. A sandal

3. A casual shoe

4. A walking shoe

1. A handbag or envelope

2. A clutch

3. A shoulder bag or brief purse

4. A tote

A BASIC WARDROBE PLAN

Coats

Basic — Neutral or basic color. Cloth, Classic style.
Fun — Neutral, basic or bright color. Patterned or textured fabric or leather.
Rain — Light, bright or neutral color. Waterproof cloth or vinyl. (Fun and Rain could the same coat.)
Jacket — Blazer, heavy sweater or car coat, depending on lifestyle and warmth desired.
Evening — Short fur jacket, stole, long coat or cape.

Basic Skirt Suit

Must be, or look like a natural fiber.
1 for winter of wool or a blend.
1 for summer of linen, cotton, silk, etc.

Basic Dress

1 or 2 of simple, classic style. Medium to dark neutral or basic color. Flat-textured, dull-surfaced fabric. Must be, or look like a natural fiber.

Occasion, After-Five Wear

Short cocktail dress. Silk, Quiana, etc. More elegant, Could be lustrous.
1 or 2 long garments — dress, pajamas, skirt and blouse, tunic with pants, etc. Cotton, silk, jersey, velveteen, etc.
1 ball gown. Elegant and memorable. Plain or elaborate, dull or shiny, according to personality and lifestyle.

Casual Dresses

2 or 3 cotton, linen, wool, etc. More detailed design or patterned fabric, geared to your personality and lifestyle. Have variety for changes of climate.

Casual Coordinates

2 or 3 skirts. For easy walking. Wool, cotton, linen, etc.
6 to 8 tops. Long and short sleeves. Blouses and knit tops of polyester, cotton, silk, etc.
3 to 4 pants. Dressy and casual. Polyester knit, wool, linen, cotton blends.
4 sweaters: 1 or 2 cardigans with long sleeves; 1 or 2 pullovers with long or short sleeves.

Pant Suit

Must be, or look like natural fiber.
1 for winter of wool or a blend.
1 for summer of linen, silk, cotton or polyester blend.

Tailored, with matching jacket and slacks. Medium to dark neutral or basic color. Flat-textured, dull-finished fabric. Avoid plaid.

Leisure, At-Home Wear

As lifestyle demands: caftans, long skirt and top, patio dress, pajamas, jumpsuit, velour jogging suit.
For gardening or cleaning: pants, shirts, tennis shoes, hat, gloves, thongs, cover-up smock or apron.
For special activities: garments for jogging, tennis, skiing, swimming, square dancing, golfing, camping, etc.

Shoes

One Neutral Color
Basic Pump
Sandal
Casual Shoe
Walking Shoe

Bags

One Neutral Color
Hand Bag or Envelope Clutch
Shoulder or Brief Purse
Tote

Jewelry

Metal — Gold or Silver
Shiny for Casual
Brushed for Dress
Pearls — Two Lengths Short and Matinee
Chains, Earrings, Pins, Bracelets, Rings

Hats

Basic Felt — Light to Medium Neutral
Straw — Neutral or Bright

Gloves

As Lifestyle Dictates
Plain Cotton, Neutral
Leather or Kid for Dress or Casual
Warm Gloves as Needed

Intimate Apparel

Bras — 2 or 3
Slips — 2 or 3
Panties — 6 pair
Hose — 6 Pairs of One Shade
Robes — 1 Warm, 1 Caftan
House Footwear Suited to Your Lifestyle

Wardrobe Basics

The backbone of every well-planned wardrobe is the *Basic Coat, Suit* and *Dress*. These should be your most expensive articles because they get more wear and therefore must be chosen carefully to be flattering, fashionable and suitable for the occasion. Because of the simplicity of the basic costume, it is important that the fabric, workmanship and fit be of the finest quality your budget will allow.

BASIC CLOTH COAT — Your coat represents your largest single expenditure and should last from two to five years. Simplicity of style and perfection of fabric, line and fit are necessary. This is the topper you'll wear over most of your wardrobe. It should have a deep armhole to be worn over suits or bulky clothes. It should be well-tailored, full length and of a modified flare, semi-shaped or straight cut rather than a closely fitted or extremely flared design. The coat may be collarless or have a shawl collar or a small collar of fabric, rather than fur or velvet trims. If there are any buttons, they should be matching or self-covered. Slit or welt pockets are preferable to patch pockets which give the coat a more casual appearance. Choose durable fabric which resists wrinkles, shine and pilling. Wool is worth paying for in terms of long-term satisfaction; it should be heavy or lightweight depending on climate. Any style that you select must strike a balance between the sporty and the dressy. Avoid heavy cuffs, unusual shapes in sleeves, contrasting belts and back flares, all of which date a fashion. Choose a neutral or basic color from your palette which harmonizes with your coloring.

FUN COATS AND RAINCOATS — These are the coats you wear to ballgames or to the grocery store and throw on for errands. We suggest a bright color to give a lift to your wardrobe, or genuine leather for a touch of casual elegance.

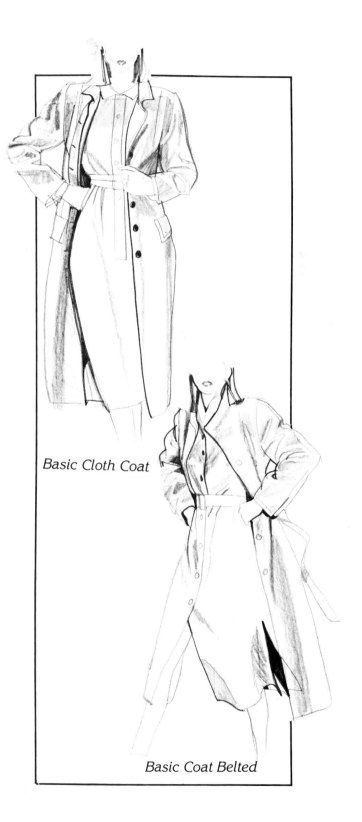

Basic Cloth Coat

Basic Coat Belted

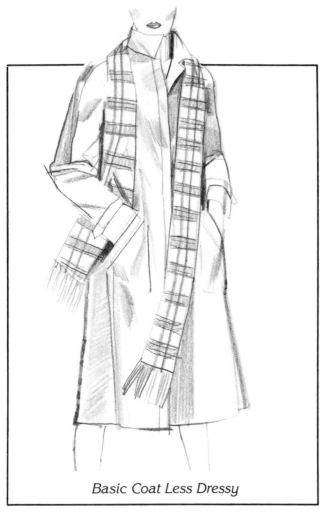

Basic Coat Less Dressy

Ultra Suede™ is a good choice, but we discourage other types of artificial leathers because they are not warm, they get stiff and can crack in cold weather and may look tacky.

EVENING WRAPS — A *long coat* may be of velveteen, wool or exotic fabrics. The need for this type of floor-length coat will be determined by your lifestyle. If you attend formal functions frequently or live in a cold metropolitan area, you could justify the purchase of a long coat.

To look good, a *cape* requires that you have a graceful carriage because it restricts your movement somewhat. Capes are most suitable for the Classic personality.

A *jacket* of velveteen, brocade, wool or a novelty fabric will serve as an evening wrap or for dressy-after five wear. A velveteen jacket will go almost anyplace.

A *stole* is a rectangular strip of fabric or fur. Depending on the fabric used, it can serve for evening or day wear. The width of the stole when draped across the shoulder should not extend below the waist in back with either a long or a short dress. To determine the proper length of a stole, fold it in half lengthwise. Held up against you with the folded edge even with your shoulders, a stole for a short dress should extend to the knees. For a long dress, it may be the same length as worn with a short dress or extend to the ankle.

Shawls are triangular. The point of the shawl should never extend below your crotch in back, especially with street-length dresses. A shawl looks best with a long dress. Wear shawls and stoles with flair, draped gracefully around the shoulders, never hugging the neck.

FUR COAT OR JACKET — A fur jacket is one of the best investments for a modern lifestyle because it can be worn with long and short dresses or pants. Fur is a status symbol. Shopping for fur calls for infinitely more care than the purchase of anything else in your wardrobe. Bargains in furs are chancy unless you are an expert who knows quality and construction. Well-made fur coats are beautifully matched and uniform in color, depth and texture. Harmonize fur to hair color, better lighter than too dark. Check areas that are subject to hard wear, such as cuffs, front closing, sleeves, back of neck and pockets. The fur should be full and thick. Make sure the fur coat you choose fits comfortably. Buy the best quality within the price range you can afford. Some furs wear better than others. Fur can make your inexpensive clothes look more expensive. Fake fur can be almost as beautiful as real fur, if of good quality, and the expense and upkeep are much less.

BLAZER — A blazer is a shaped jacket which comes to the crotch in front. It will dress up any pair of pants, even jeans. Choose a lightweight linen-type of fabric for summer wear and heavier fabric for winters.

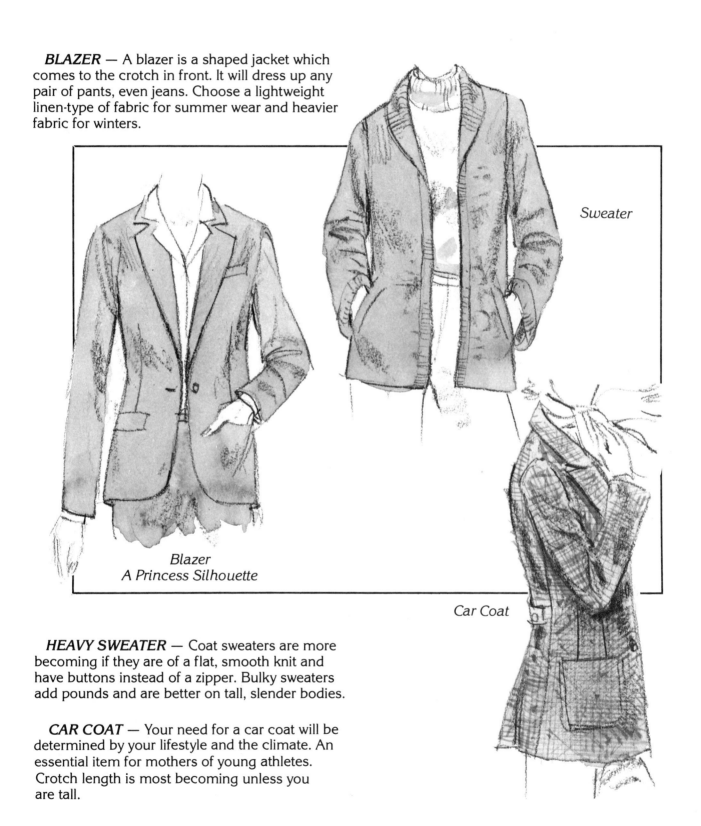

Sweater

Blazer
A Princess Silhouette

Car Coat

HEAVY SWEATER — Coat sweaters are more becoming if they are of a flat, smooth knit and have buttons instead of a zipper. Bulky sweaters add pounds and are better on tall, slender bodies.

CAR COAT — Your need for a car coat will be determined by your lifestyle and the climate. An essential item for mothers of young athletes. Crotch length is most becoming unless you are tall.

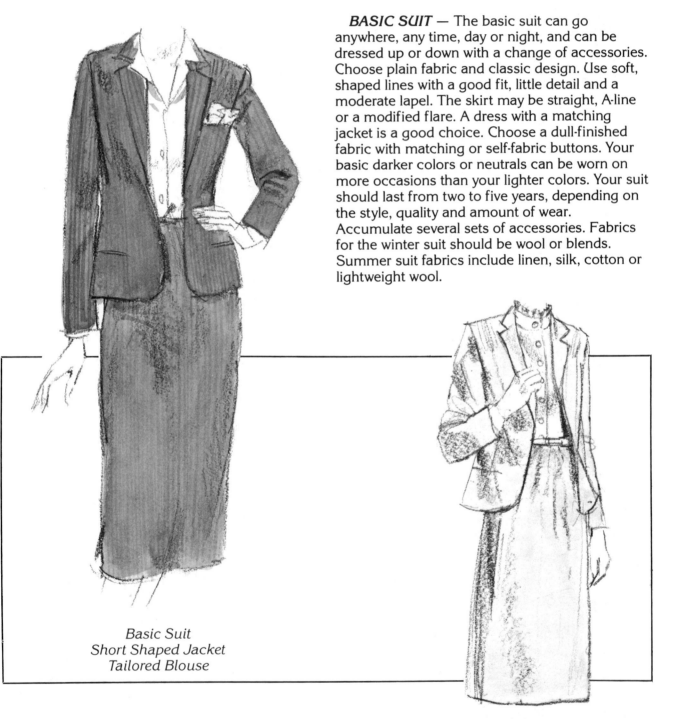

BASIC SUIT — The basic suit can go anywhere, any time, day or night, and can be dressed up or down with a change of accessories. Choose plain fabric and classic design. Use soft, shaped lines with a good fit, little detail and a moderate lapel. The skirt may be straight, A-line or a modified flare. A dress with a matching jacket is a good choice. Choose a dull-finished fabric with matching or self-fabric buttons. Your basic darker colors or neutrals can be worn on more occasions than your lighter colors. Your suit should last from two to five years, depending on the style, quality and amount of wear. Accumulate several sets of accessories. Fabrics for the winter suit should be wool or blends. Summer suit fabrics include linen, silk, cotton or lightweight wool.

Basic Suit
Short Shaped Jacket
Tailored Blouse

Basic Suit
Short Shaped Jacket
Feminine Blouse

BASIC DRESS — A basic dress is street length and of simple, classic style with long sleeves. It should be comfortably cut, well fitted and easy to slip into. The skirt should have walking and sitting room, and the neckline should be modest. You should be able to wear this basic dress day or night, dressing it up or down by using some of the same accessories acquired for your basic suit. This is the dress to wear when you don't know what to wear. It will take you to breakfast, lunch, dinner, theatre, weddings, parties, etc. The basic dress should be of a flat-textured, dull-surfaced fabric. It must be of, or look like a natural fiber. Choose your most becoming medium to dark neutral or basic color. You will need one for cold climate and one for warm weather.

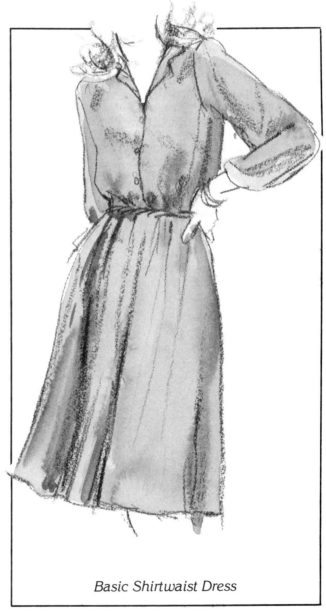

Basic Shirtwaist Dress

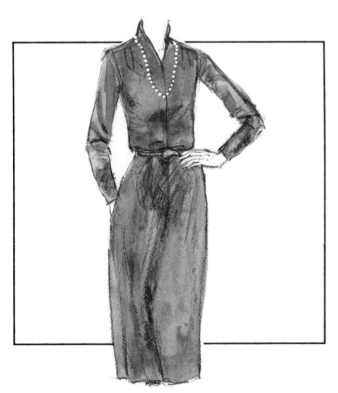

Basic Dress

OCCASION, AFTER-FIVE DRESS — This dress is street length or longer. It might have a handkerchief or novelty hem. The after-five special occasion dress may be elegant — high fashion, or a striking understatement in costly fabric. Choose a modest or decollete neckline depending on your personality. Your lifestyle will determine if you need this dress. *Long* — The need for a floor-length after-five dressy garment will be determined by where you live, your social circle and current fashion. Long fashions fade in and out of your wardrobe. Pajamas, jumpsuits, tunic pantsets, long skirts, etc. are popular on a

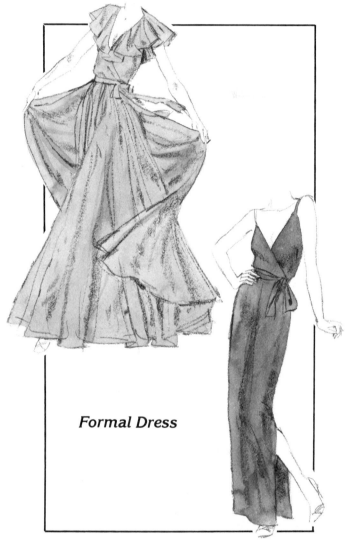

Formal Dress

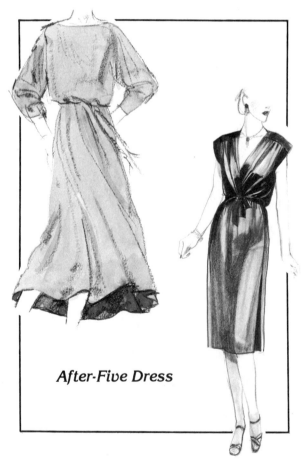

After-Five Dress

three- to five-year fashion cycle. Keep a few, they'll come back. *Ball Gowns* — Only if your lifestyle warrants such an expenditure should you spend a great deal on this type of dress. Most women need only one. If your big annual affair is with the same group of friends each year, you would be wise to choose a less elaborate or memorable gown.

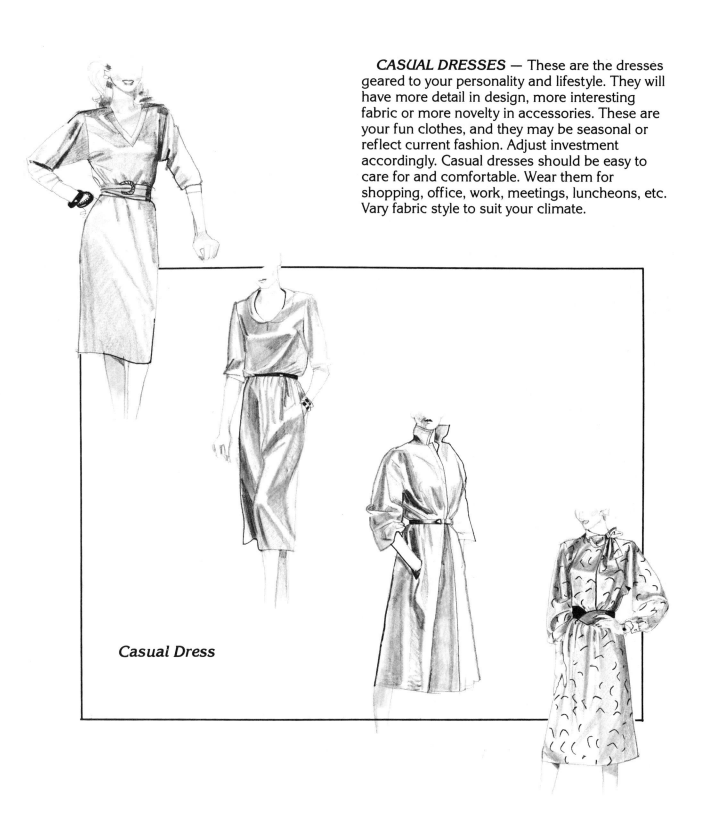

CASUAL DRESSES — These are the dresses geared to your personality and lifestyle. They will have more detail in design, more interesting fabric or more novelty in accessories. These are your fun clothes, and they may be seasonal or reflect current fashion. Adjust investment accordingly. Casual dresses should be easy to care for and comfortable. Wear them for shopping, office, work, meetings, luncheons, etc. Vary fabric style to suit your climate.

Casual Dress

CASUAL COORDINATES — These are the clothes you live in and which will make or break your reputation as a well-dressed, put-together woman. Casual coordinates can be divided into two categories: the clothes you wear in public and the clothes you wear around the house. This is where most women skimp, fail to use imagination and do not really meet their lifestyle needs. With casual coordinates you can enjoy fads and inexpensive extras which will add flair and express your personality. Contrasting tops and bottoms will cut you in half and always give a more casual appearance. Pieces which match or coordinate, carrying one color into both pieces (with print and plain), give a more organized, meant-to-go-together appearance. Tops and bottoms of the same color will make you appear taller and slimmer. Choose medium to dark colors if you are overweight.

Casual coordinates for public appearance should be, or look like a natural fiber. They could be washable or dry cleanable. Slacks should be creased and of a length to take a higher heel, which makes pants look dressier. Skirts that can be worn with a heel and a dressier blouse give you a more classic, dressed-up look.

PANT SUITS — Every woman needs at least one tailored pant suit. A pant suit can be accessorized with hat and gloves if desired for a very put-together look. You could wear a pant suit anywhere in the world in metropolitan areas and be considered well dressed. The jacket and pants should be of matching or coordinated fabric, which is, or looks like a natural fiber. A blend of natural and synthetic fibers gives added wrinkle resistance while retaining the comfort of the natural fiber.

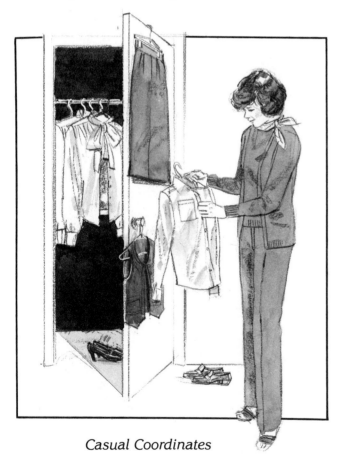

Casual Coordinates

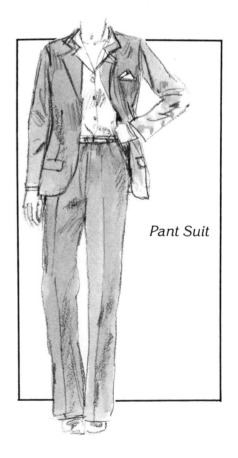

Pant Suit

LEISURE, AT-HOME WEAR — Clothes for wear around the house must be washable and of a length for comfortable shoes. If you want to get out of character, this is the place to do it, on your own time. Wear bright muumuus or exotic prints with bare feet. Relax in an elegant velour jogging suit. Greet your family in a comfortable caftan. Look good at home for the most important people in your life.

By careful planning and utilizing this basic wardrobe plan you can be the best dressed woman in your group and yet spend less money. The only thing left to add is your flair with accessories.

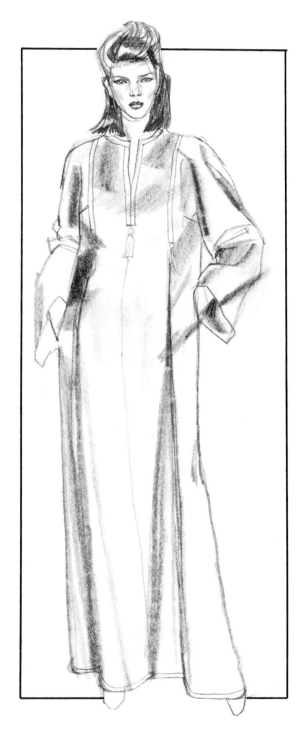

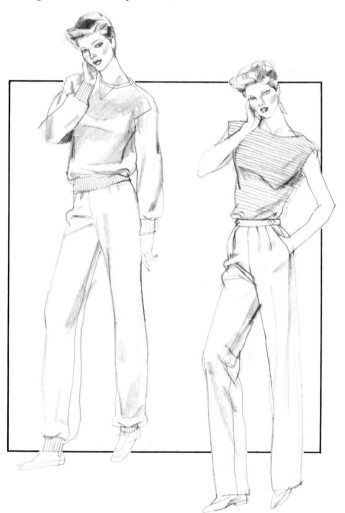

159

Spending Your Fashion Dollar Wisely

Should you do your shopping at a big department store or a small shop? Each has its buyer's taste coincides with your taste and your pocketbook. Learn to recognize the stores which specialize in good taste, and look for fashion there. Some stores specialize in volume merchandising and can offer good buys in basic necessities such as hose, underwear, accessories, etc. Consider style and wearability in relation to the original and upkeep costs. Know the size you require for comfort and wearability, but recognize that size varies with different manufacturers. advantages and problems. The difference between a department store and a small shop boils down to the fact that in a small shop, the owner or manager is running the business and has a big stake in keeping you well-satisfied and coming back, while the average department store clerk is holding down a job, and one customer is as good as another in her sales book. Your choice is determined by where you get the best service and the best buys for your money.

Time is money in shopping. Find the store that specializes in the kind of merchandise which is suited to your individual needs and where the

Department Stores

Quantity buying usually makes prices more reasonable at department stores. Because plenty of floor space is available, a wider selection of styles is offered. Returns are easily and pleasantly made. A reputable department store stands behind its merchandise. Defective garments will be returned to the manufacturer. Returns for other reasons are made with a minimum of fuss and bother. They all buy from the same sources, so they may carry the same merchandise.

Small Shops

Small shops may offer specialized service, and the atmosphere is often pleasant and unique. In a well-run small shop, you get personal attention. A wise shop owner is interested in making a sale but also in gaining a steady customer. Small shops usually specialize in a certain type of clothing keyed to a particular type of woman. It is easy to exchange or get credit for returned merchandise, but often difficult to get cash refunds. Always ask about store policy before making your purchase.

Labels

Read labels carefully for information as to the fiber content and percentage, shrinkage, colorfastness, type of finish and care required. Each manufacturer (cutter) has a particular body type in mind when he makes his clothes. All of his garments are cut from the same master pattern. For example, if one size 10 Evan Picone™ jacket fits you perfectly, chances are that all Evan Picone™ jackets of the same size will fit you. Find the cutter who has you in mind.

Quality

Plan the purchase of more costly garments, such as suits and coats, for different times. Buy the best you can afford. Never count the cost of the garment or accessory. It is the cost-per-wearing that counts. Quality is often economy. Buy more non-seasonal than seasonal clothing. Keep to a neutral or basic color for more expensive accessories and outer garments such as coats and suits. A neutral color in an inexpensive dress may make it appear more costly. Avoid too much decoration on an inexpensive dress; it looks cheap. The lowest-priced garment is not always the most economical. Evaluate in terms of good design, lasting fashion, durability of fabric, ease of care and suitability to you and your way of life.

Buying At Sales

If it is service you want, forget about sale buying. If you know merchandise and are familiar with name-brand manufacturers, a sale can be a worthwhile experience. Be aware that many stores import inferior or old merchandise for a sale. There are two ways to shop at a clearance sale — one, early for the cream; two, late for the drippings. Beware of wholesale buying unless your connections are very good indeed.

Spending Your Money Where It Counts

Learn to judge fashion. Study fashion magazines, learn to discriminate between fashions that are well-designed, functional, beautiful, and becoming and those that are merely "new and different." Clothes, their cost or source, are not as important as what you do with them. A little flair and good accessories can make a mediocre garment smashing. Buy clothes for your lifestyle. Spend your money where you spend your time.

Fashion Rules To Follow

☐ Be vain about your good points — vain enough to make the most of them.
☐ Keep your figure challenges a secret by choosing clothes to conceal them.
☐ Know your lines, the fashion lines that flatter *you*. Use color to flattering advantage.
☐ Dress to suit the occasion. If you are not sure, wear something so simple that you won't feel either over- or under-done.
☐ Keep within your budget. It's not how much you spend, but how wisely and tastefully you spend that makes you well dressed.
☐ Use accessories wisely. They can make a basic dress or suit change, and change, and change.
☐ Remember that *ready-to-wear* is a term that should apply to everything you own. Always have your clothes clean and well pressed. Every appearance is an important one.

Shopping Laws

1. Shop alone when you want to keep your mind on what you are doing. When you have no specific shopping chore in mind, take a friend. Make sure she is a good friend and won't talk you into something that isn't right for you. Invite your husband, father or best beau to go shopping with you. Chances are you will buy something more costly and of better quality than you would have bought by yourself.

2. You could leave your checkbook and charge plate home, but that's no fun. You will never achieve personal style until you develop discipline. Do more looking and less buying. Looking keeps you abreast of fashion trends and passing fads.

3. Dress well when shopping to gain respect from salespeople. When shopping for dress shoes, wear a dress; for pant shoes, wear pants.

4. Forget all preconceived ideas about color.

5. Decide which neutral you want to work with.

6. Decide what you really need, putting first things first. Use your priority shopping list to control impulse buying and develop sales resistance.

7. Shop for your colors in your own season.

8. When buying a suit, dress, bra, girdle, swimwear, etc., bend, stretch and sit in them.

9. Before buying ask yourself: Is this suitable for *my* lifestyle, will I get enough use out of it, and what will it cost in terms of money or time to keep it clean?

10. Consider each purchase in this order: *Size. Color. Line. Texture. Fit. Personality.*

11. If you are not happy, excited and confident about your purchase, *don't buy it!*

Everyone has a wardrobe budget — the amount in it is merely relative. By utilizing a wardrobe plan when shopping, you will stretch your clothing budget to fit your needs.

Looking Good While Traveling Light

What you take when you travel depends on where you are going. *Eliminate!* We tend to pack everything in sight, and then we are weighted down with luggage containing clothes we will never wear. The charge for overweight is prohibitive on the return trip. In foreign countries you will be handling your own baggage. Take only what you can carry. Even in countries where porter service is available, waiting for help could result in missed connections. Use soft-sided luggage as it withstands impact better and will hold more.

When you travel you do not see the same people. You may tire of wearing the same thing, but the people will never see you again. If you are on tour, people don't mind seeing you in the same thing if you always look good, and *you will* look better than they do because you are not tired from carrying all that luggage or frustrated from trying to decide what to wear.

Neutral colors are fine for short trips but not for long, tiring journeys. If your travel clothes are in a neutral, plan to have a bright touch near the face. Plan your wardrobe around your most becoming medium to dark colors. Fabric of moderate texture with a dull finish shows fewer wrinkles and less soil and it goes more places. Polyester is a joy to take abroad if you don't mind being recognized as an American. The prices go up if they recognize you. Choose fabrics that have a look of natural fiber, though they may be made of synthetics. Blends give you the best of both worlds. Polyester, nylon and acrylic have no wickability. This means that they do not absorb body moisture or breathe as do the natural fibers. If your destination is a tropical climate, you had best make do with the wrinkles and choose natural fibers. There are fine imported cottons which do not wrinkle very much, and woolens so sheer, wrinkle-resistant and cool that they are used for hot-weather uniforms by the military.

Basic Wardrobe Combinations To Suit Travel Needs

A tailored jacket with skirt and/or pants — You may add as many blouses and tops as desired. If you are short and wish to wear a skirt and pants with the same jacket, the jacket should be short enough to balance your figure. Pants are accepted wear for women in every cosmopolitan center in the world. In some parts of the city, in some churches and in provincial towns, however, you will be more comfortable in a skirt.

The dress with a jacket or matching sweater is a versatile addition to a travel wardrobe. Have coordinated skirts, pants and blouses. A lightweight cardigan sweater is essential.

A knit dress or knit separates are easy to care for. They wear well, roll up for packing and do not wrinkle. Have them basic enough to dress up or down. Lightweight polyester can be rinsed out at night to dry by morning. Plan on washing only your lightweight blouses and tops or you may be packing or wearing them wet.

The all-weather coat for rain or shine should be an in-between style to wear over casual or dressy clothes. Any fabric can be waterproofed. Ultra Suede™ is incomparably elegant and practical for travel in cooler climates.

Take three sets of *underclothes*, the one you are wearing, one change and one drying.

Bed and loungewear should be versatile. One nightie will suffice. A caftan or muumuu can double as a robe or loungewear. Add soft, packable slippers.

Accessories

Shoes — One comfortable pair of low-heeled walking shoes and one pair with a higher heel for dress. Other types to suit your itinerary.

Gloves — One pair to wear with the basic coat or suit if warmth is a consideration.

Hat or scarf — Something to protect hair from sun, wind and rain.

Bags — One large tote bag, one clutch for dress or evening wear.

Jewelry — Basic, brushed and shiny, gold or silver, a watch, pearls. Coordinate so you have something for both sport and dress.

Necessities — Cosmetics, skin and hair care products, medicine, etc. Be sure to use only plastic bottles with tight, screw-on lids. Take a travel clock if you have a time schedule.

How You Travel Determines What You Wear

By Plane — Dress nicely but comfortably in a basic dress with jacket or coat, basic suit or pant suit. Choose a fabric which will not show wrinkles or become rump-sprung. Take stretch slipper-socks for comfort on a long flight if altitude tends to make your feet swell. Put on a comfortable girdle or none at all. Have clothes styled not to require the restriction of a girdle. Use a train case or tote bag to carry beauty aids, books, sweater, slippers or whatever you need at hand.

By Train — Wear pant sets or coordinates that are comfortable. Take a train case or tote bag for beauty aids, toilet articles, night clothes, sweater, slippers, books, knitting, sewing, etc.

By Ship — Casual clothes are needed for daytime activities and sightseeing trips ashore. An all-weather coat is essential for warmth or protection from tropical storms. Take glad rags for the gala after-dark doings that make an ocean voyage so glamorous. Wear walking shoes for trips ashore and dress shoes for evening. Play shoes are good for doing your thing on board during the daytime cruises. A casual wrap or sweater will protect against a chilly ocean breeze.

By Bus or Auto — Comfort is the criterion in choosing clothes for a bus or auto trip. Think twice about slacks. They can be uncomfortable if you are sitting all day, and they are warmer than a skirt. Consider as an alternative for slacks an easy skirt with cool tops and short jackets or sweaters. An easy-fitting dress in a knit, seersucker or jersey is a good choice. For a long trip where you are eating in restaurants, a well-coordinated outfit is best. For short car trips, jeans with coordinated blouses or sweaters are suitable. Flat-heeled shoes are best if you are driving, but keep some heels handy. You can switch into them and dress up your outfit to visit a restaurant or to make a grand entrance at journey's end. Neutrals do nothing for tired people. Color near the face will give you a lift.

Wherever you travel remember that vacation is no time to relax the standards you have set for your appearance. Time your haircuts, permanents, and tints to have your hair just right for your trip. Plan your wardrobe as if you were planning a trip. Even if you are not, we believe that if you prepare for an event, it will happen. Plan around one neutral color so that you have the shoes, bags and accessories to harmonize, then add the clothes to complete a compact wardrobe grouping that will take you anywhere.

Whatever you wear, you'll enjoy your trip more if you are comfortably dressed and know you look your best. Nowhere in your wardrobe plan is it more important to use all your new-found knowledge.

CHAPTER TEN

Accessories

YOUR PERSONAL STYLE – ADDING FLAIR

The choice of accessories is a matter of good taste. Good taste is the ability to recognize and enjoy what is beautiful and excellent, a sense of what is harmonious, appropriate and socially proper. Some people are born with a sense of good taste, while others have to acquire it. Many things influence what is considered good taste — where you live, your culture, age and lifestyle. What is proper in New York City, for example, is not necessarily good in Southern California.

Accessories refer to everything except the garment, and they play an important part in any wardrobe. They include shoes, handbags, gloves, scarves, furs, belts, hats, jewelry, eyeglasses, flowers, trims and nail polish. It takes time, good planning and a lot of imagination to accessorize your clothes properly. Choose accessories that harmonize with each other and that can be worn with more than one outfit. All accessories should be purchased with *your* personality in mind. Be a collector of good accessories and choose them for lasting value. Keep up and have fun with the constantly changing fads, but invest the money in the timeless classics for the basis of your accessory collection — quality leather, good metals and jewelry.

Like the frosting on the cake, accessories are either fresh, smooth and inviting or better omitted. Accessories do not need to match, but they should harmonize. In assembling a costume, you are creating a work of art. You must have one center of interest. Other points of interest must be subordinate to that one. Too many points of interest weaken and cheapen the whole look. Strive for simplicity.

When choosing accessories, if in doubt — don't!

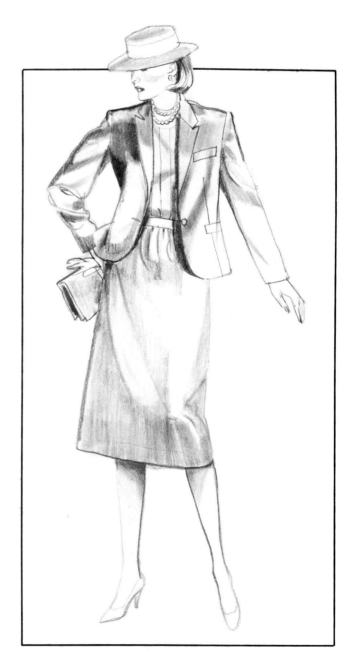

165

Shoes

In putting together a good wardrobe, shoes present the greatest challenge because of the difficulty in obtaining good style, good fit and good color combined in the same shoe.

More than any accessory, shoes can make or break your total fashion look. The shoe must harmonize in feeling with the garment. Dainty, strappy, thin-soled, narrow-heeled shoes belong with longer, more delicate dreses. Thicker-soled, sturdier-heeled, more substantial shoes go with heavier fabrics, sportier clothes or with shorter skirts.

Shoes of a neutral color are most basic and are your best investment. The shoe should be the same *color* or *value* as the hemline or *darker*. The eye will always go to the lightest part of the costume. Light-colored shoes — white or bone — should be worn only with clothing of the same or lighter value, pastels or a light-colored print. A brighter shoe, such as red, should be worn with a garment which has red in it or you must bring the eye back up to the face with a blouse, sweater or scarf of red.

Wear a dress when shopping for dress shoes and pants when buying pant shoes.

Calf leather is most basic. Kid is very dressy, fragile and expensive. Suede goes with most everything nine months of the year, but not with summertime cottons. Suede shoes are bulky and will make your feet look bigger.

Patent leather is considered a summertime shoe but is worn year round in warm climates.

Lamé makes a wintertime, holiday, very dressy shoe and bag. Lamé looks best in strappy sandals and clutch bags. Reptile skin, because of its heavy texture, is best suited for Autumns and Winters. If texture is desired by Springs and Summers, ostrich, eel or snake is a better choice.

Your basic wardrobe should include four styles of shoes, all in the same neutral color. See the chart of neutrals for your season on pages 8-25.

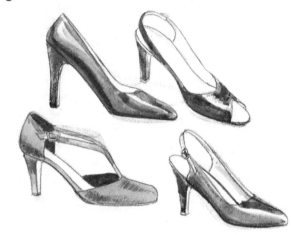

Pump — If you could have only one pair of dress shoes to go with all of your skirts, dresses and suits, it should be a pump. A classic pump is becoming on all legs. The pump with toe and/or heel out is more romantic and feminine. The pump with a strap is best on a slim leg. The T-strap shoe looks best on the narrow foot and slim leg.

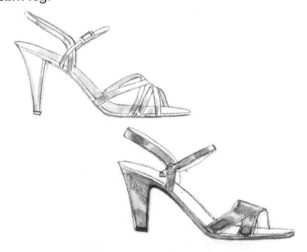

Sandal — The more foot and the less shoe, the dressier the sandal. The broad-strapped, thicker-soled sandal is versatile and can be worn with dresses or pants, but it is more casual.

Casual Shoe — The casual shoe with a walking heel will compliment your pant outfits or your casual daytime dresses or skirts. You might need one pair of pant shoes with a higher vamp for your tailored winter slack suit. If the vamp is not too high, the sides are cut lower and the leg is slim, this shoe will also team with sporty dresses or skirts.

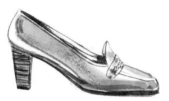

Walking Shoe — This is the shoe you live in for your casual, everyday life. It should have a lower heel and be comfortable enough for hours of walking.

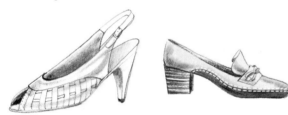

After you have acquired your four basic shoes, add as many of these extras as your budget will allow.

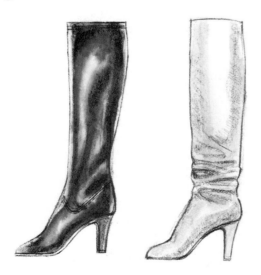

Boots — Boots are extra except in cold climates. Choose simple, classic, quality boots with a sensible walking heel. Choose a style to fit your personality and lifestyle. Boots may feel good in the store, but after you have worn them around your house for an hour, on the carpet, they may feel sloppy big and need to be exchanged. A large calf would need a crushed, stovepipe-style boot. The skirt should cover the top of the boot if it is calf length.

Espadrille — Very popular and comfortable for a casual lifestyle. Available in many colors and materials, espadrilles are great when worn with casual skirts and pants.

Backless Slides, Wooden Platform Heels Or Clogs — Made popular by the younger girls, they are comfortable to stand in, terrible to walk in and look horrible from the back, especially if your foot is large and your leg is full.

Thong Sandals — Thongs belong at a beach or resort or around the house. They are more attractive if the toes are controlled.

Fads and Fancies — If you have shoes in your closet which are miserably uncomfortable but absolutely adorable, you are a shoeaholic. If you are in search of a beautiful, fashionable, comfortable shoe, forget it; it's a dream — if the shoe fits, it's ugly!

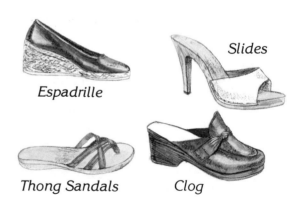

Espadrille

Slides

Thong Sandals

Clog

Bags

Economize in any area of your wardrobe but not in your handbag. Buy the best you can afford in a simple design, take good care of it and you will carry it for years. Neutral bags are basic and are your best investment. Your bag should be the same color or value as your shoes or lighter. The bag does not need to match your shoes, but it should harmonize. Your everyday bag should be roomy enough to hold all the paraphernalia you normally carry, but it must be in proportion to your size. Small women love big bags, although they are overpowered by them.

Choose slim gussets for a slimmer look in your hip and thigh area. A gusset is the inset piece at each end which controls how wide the bag can spread. Colored shoes add spice to your wardrobe, but you do not need to buy a matching colored bag. Use your neutral leather, fabric or straw bag. Store bags by filling them with tissue paper and protecting them from dust.

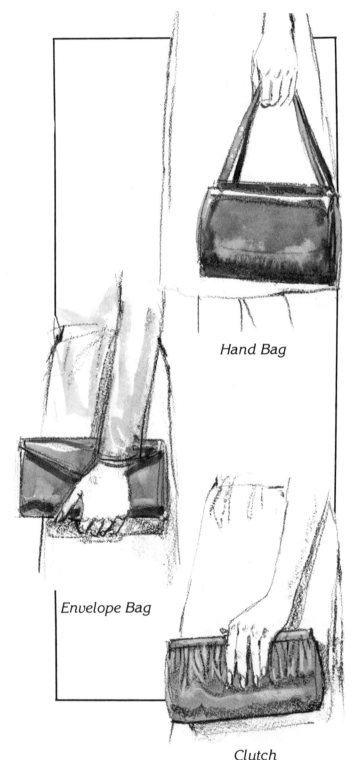

Hand Bag

Envelope Bag

Clutch

Your basic wardrobe should include four types of bag, all in the same color.

Handbags are used with dresses or suits, but not with pants. The bottom of the bag should not extend much below the hemline.

An *envelope bag* is more versatile and has currently taken the place of the handbag. It looks equally good with skirts or pants. The only trouble with an envelope bag is that it does not hold much. It is awkward and bulky when shopping, but looks super if you can bring yourself to leave all your junk at home.

A *clutch* is a small bag, usually soft, with the clasp at the top. You may really be insecure with this one because all it will hold is a hanky, a lipstick and a credit card. A clutch is a dressy bag to wear with sandals. You will eventually have several in your essential neutral colors. Buy good quality, very simple — they never go out of style.

A *brief purse* is a good choice for a professional woman if she hauls around papers and appointment books. It functions as a briefcase but is still considered a purse. One should never carry a briefcase and a purse. If you need to carry a briefcase and are going out to lunch, tuck a clutch or envelope bag inside.

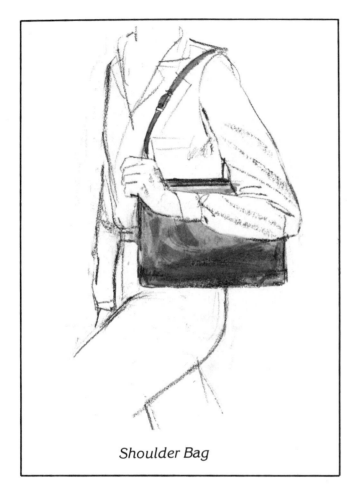

Shoulder Bag

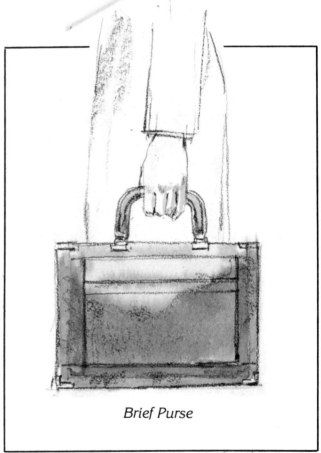

Brief Purse

Shoulder bags go best with pants or sport outfits. Avoid getting your shoulder bag too long or too wide. The shoulder bag will ride more comfortably and securely near your waistline so that your hand can rest either on the top or on the bottom. The bottom of the bag should never hang any lower than the hip line. A local shoemaker can shorten the strap. The shoulder bag is considered an everyday, run-around accessory. When worn with your better clothes, the strap distorts the shoulder line.

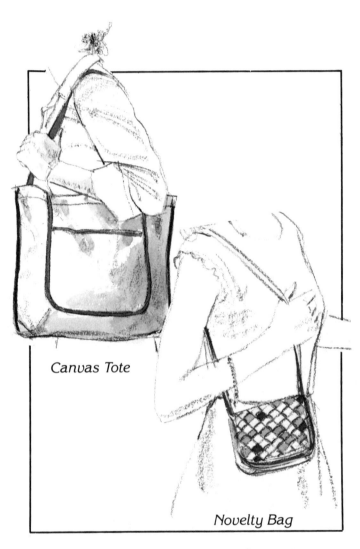

Canvas Tote

Novelty Bag

A *tote* is like a small suitcase, ideal for the woman who likes to carry everything she owns with her. It is great for travel in leather or canvas. The tote is a stylish substitute for a diaper bag and is indispensable at a beach or resort. Straw totes are fun, but expect only one or two summer seasons' wear because they are fragile.

Novelty bags are one kind of item in which you can express your artsy-craftsy talents or indulge your whimsy. Any novelty bag is a short-lived investment. You actually need only four basic bags, but try to tell that to a purse-aholic.

Hosiery

Skin-tone hose are most becoming and are always your best choice. Very dark, very light or novelty hose call attention to the legs. That is fine if your legs are your best feature. Dark, sheer hosiery is an evening look and when worn, hem and shoes should match. Light or white hose become the center of interest of any costume unless the hemline and shoe are of the same tone. Light hose are not flattering to the leg. Opaque hose in dark shades, neutrals or colors give a sporty look and should match the hem and shoes. Opaque hose are only good on young, long, slender legs. Sheer hose with novelty designs are a regularly recurring fad. Sparkles are for evening.

Winter wears light to dark gray, taupe-tone, coffee or rose-tone beige. She may also wear gray, navy or black in the wintertime if matched to the shoe and hem. Black and navy hose are for evening wear. The Winter woman should not wear cinnamon or golden suntans.

Summer wears taupe in light tones, rose-beige, light gray and navy. No golden suntans, cinnamon or black.

Spring wears nude tones, ivory, light golden-beige, light suntan and light navy. Avoid dark brown, cinnamon or black.

Autumn wears golden tones, suntans, browns and cinnamons. No taupe or gray tones.

Eyewear

Eyeglasses are more than just another accessory — they are vital to your health and

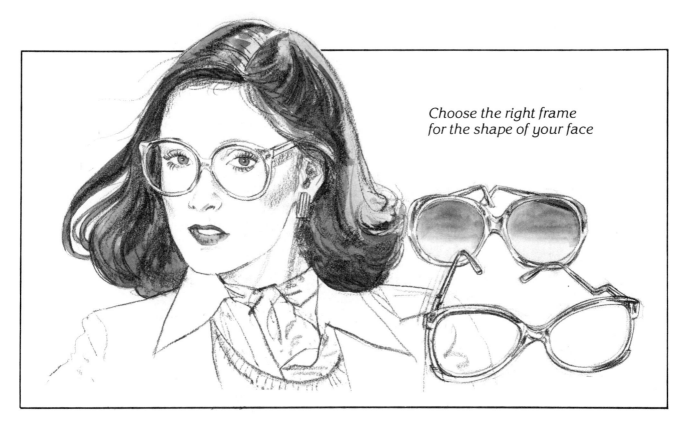

*Choose the right frame
for the shape of your face*

often to how effectively you deal with the world. Whether or not you wear glasses all the time, they are part of you and should complement your appearance and exemplify your personality and lifestyle.

Glasses today are such becoming fashion items that some people look better with than without them. Regardless of whether you look better with or without glasses, you should have more than one pair. When shopping for eyewear, take someone along who can be objective and helpful. Involved in your choices are:

Fashion — This refers to the eyeglasses themselves, the material of which they are constructed, the design and size of the frame, color of the lens, and shape of the earpiece. Be alert to changing fashion. You might need to change glasses to stay in style more frequently

than you need to change your prescription.

Shape — The shape of the frame is determined by your facial contours and features. The rules of shape are general, modified according to each individual. To begin with, you need to be aware that different shapes of frames are available in different sizes. Then remember: The size of your face determines the size of the frame. Don't let your glasses wear you, which they will appear to do if the frames are too large. On the other hand, frames that are too small will cause your total image to loose impact.

Lifestyle — Classify your lifestyle and select eyewear accordingly. Are you a sophisticated, conservative, casual or high-fashion type? The latest Pierre Cardin frames might be smashing, but will they wear you? Delicate metal frames can be very flattering, but how will they survive your rough treatment? Are you an avant-garde artist wearing granny glasses?

If your health insurance offers an arrangement for cut-rate eyewear, you should shop at several eyewear specialty stores to acquaint yourself with what is new and to establish your taste in current fashion. Then check to see if your outlet can supply the same glasses. This is really no time to economize. You need quality, but the appearance is equally important. Use the same care you would in shopping for a plastic surgeon. For some people, eyewear is a permanent facial detail.

SUNGLASSES — If you wear glasses all the time, we discourage your trying to combine your regular glasses and sunglasses into the same eyewear by using photo-sensitive lenses. Light-sensitive lenses often do not darken enough for strong sunlight outdoors, while they do not lighten enough inside, either. And the latter is important: People need to see your eyes if you are going to establish rapport.

Sunglasses are a fashion item. They should follow the same general rules that we've set out for other eyewear, but they can be fun, large and

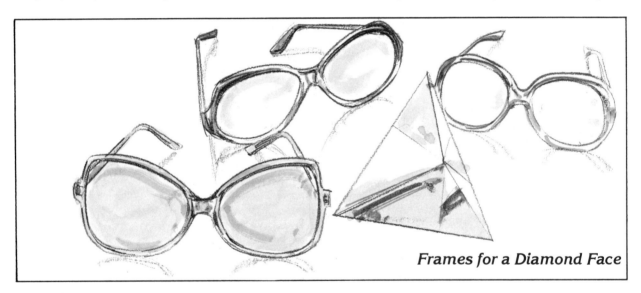

Frames for a Diamond Face

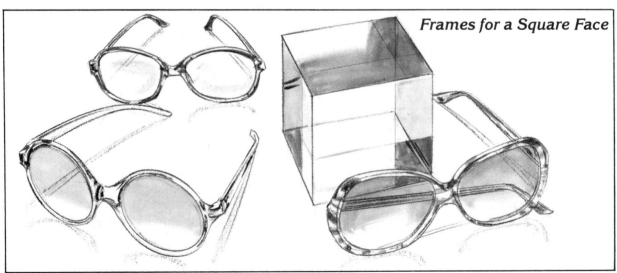

Frames for a Square Face

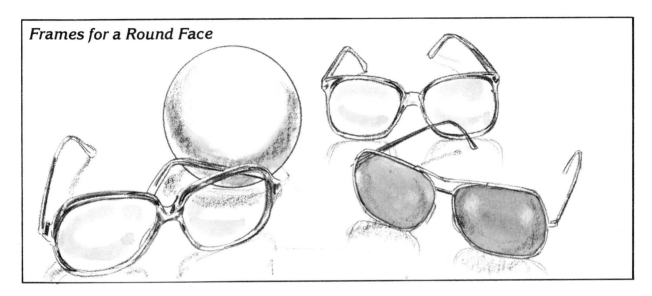

Frames for a Round Face

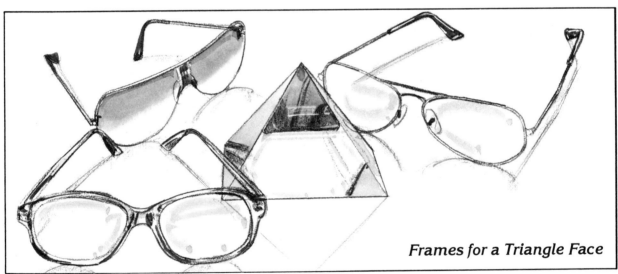

Frames for a Triangle Face

extreme — real trendy! The lenses should harmonize with your eye color and the colors of your season.

FRAMES — Frames should be as wide as the widest part of your face and in proportion to the shape and size of your face. Glasses should lift your face by having an upward line or curve on the upper frame. For good balance your eye should be in the center of the frame or lens. The lower frame should not repeat but complement your cheek and jawline. This means that you should not put round frames on a round face or square frames on a square face. The round face could wear a rounded square, and the square face a squared round.

Choose a high, slender or rounded bridge for a small nose; a low, thick or straight bridge is more becoming for a long nose.

Plastic frames should blend with your complexion and hair coloring. Winters wear charcoal-brown, gray-blues, or gray if they have gray hair. Summers look good in rose-browns, blue-grays, and gray with gray hair. Springs wear medium to light warm golden-browns and light gray when their hair is gray. Autumns look best in warm brown to red-browns (tortoise shell), and grayed brown or light gray with gray hair. Metal frames or trims should use the metal of your season — silver for Winters and Summers, and gold for Springs and Autumns.

Contact Lenses

If you wear contact lenses, the smoked lenses are best. They do not distort your eye color, yet they can be seen when dropped. Avoid colored contact lenses unless they closely match the color of your eyes to prevent an artificial look. This is no time to get baby-blue eyes — even if you have always wanted them. For sunglasses, only ground glass of good quality should be worn over contacts.

Tinted Lenses

For everyday glasses, if you decide to tint your lenses, the degree of shading should be very light, from one-half to one point of color at the top to nothing — that is, perfectly clear — at the bottom.

Winters who shade their glasses at the top would find gray or gray-blue the most effective color.

Summers can best use blue, gray or mauve.

Springs look good with a very delicate, soft brown or soft blue-gray at the top. Be careful to get only one point or less of color.

Autumns should wear from one-half to one point of light, soft brown at the top of the lenses. If they are too dark, your eyes will look tired.

You might consider adding a soft tint at the lower outside corner of the lenses — a peach

flesh tone for Springs and Autumns and a rose flesh tone for Winters and Summers. This is a marvelous device to add color to pale or sallow skin. Women who have tried it have found that no one realizes that there is color in the lenses. You don't have to wait for new glasses. If you wear plastic lenses, a tint can be added now.

If people cannot see your eyes through your colored lenses, then there is too much color in them. If the lenses are made of plastic, the color can be changed, and you should do so. People must see your eyes — they provide an important, ever-sensitive signpost to your thoughts, ideas and feelings.

The glasses you wear can do more than help you see better. They should enhance your appearance and indicate the kind of person you are and the sort of life you lead.

Add Flair

Belts — You may want to have a leather belt ½ (1 cm) to ¾ (2 cm) inch wide in a neutral color to wear with skirts and pants when the blouse is

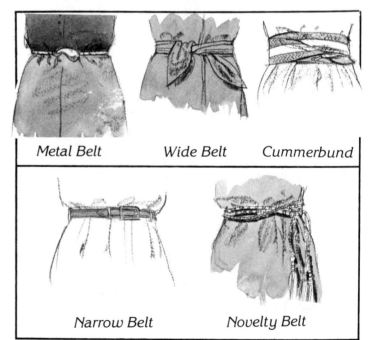

Metal Belt   Wide Belt   Cummerbund

Narrow Belt   Novelty Belt

tucked in. For a dressier look, you may add a gold or silver belt in the metal of your season to give the waistline a finished, dressy look.

Thicker waistlines should wear belts of the same fabric or color. A diminishing trick for some thick waistlines is to wear a cummerbund. It takes off inches. Novelty belts in an endless variety add interest to the costume if your waistline can tolerate the attention.

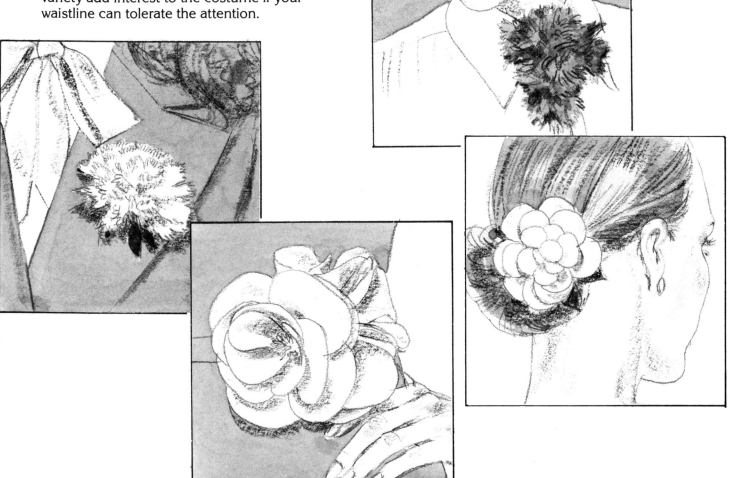

Flowers — Use flowers for lapels of dresses or suits, or at the waist of a more formal dress. A Dramatic or Romantic personality can wear a flower in the hair very successfully. Flowers add flair to your summer wardrobe. Flowers of unrealistic colors, such as a blue rose, must match the color of the garment and are more dressy. Artificial flowers of realistic color do not have to match the garment. A good choice for a Winter is a red or white carnation or a bunch of violets. A pink carnation or a rose is right for a Summer, peach or yellow rose or daisies for a Spring. Asters, chrysanthemums or yellow daisies are best for Autumn. Flower stems should be worn pointing down, as they grow. To keep your artificial flowers fresh, store them in a shoe box.

Gloves — Gloves were originally worn to keep the hands warm and clean, but they are no longer considered absolutely necessary for a well-dressed look. A good basic glove is of cloth or leather and has no trim; it can be worn with almost everything. You should own one or two pairs in your neutral colors. The best length would be a short glove that covers the wrist bone.

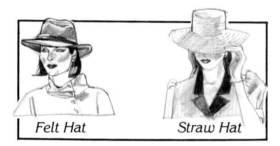

Felt Hat   *Straw Hat*

Hats — Hats are chic, fun and fashionable. If you like them, wear them. A hat will dress up any outfit. Your hat should be the same color as your collar line, lighter or brighter. Always stand up when buying a hat in order to get the overall effect. Study it from all angles. The crown should be as wide as the widest part of the face. The brim should be no wider than the shoulders. Felt is worn in the wintertime, straw in the summer. A beach or sun hat is indispensable.

Handkerchiefs — A handkerchief symbolizes your feminity. A monogrammed hanky should bear the initial of your first name. A hanky peeking from a pocket can perk up a suit.

Scarves — Scarves are fads which resurface about every other year. They add color to the face, give a sophisticated air to the overall look and help a long neck. On the other hand, if you have a short neck you can still wear them, but choose narrow, lighter-weight scarves. Shiny, firmly woven scarves are for casual sportswear. A dull, soft scarf is dressier.

Allow an extra five minutes to tie your scarf and then secure it with one or two glass-headed straight pins. Safety pins will tear a scarf.

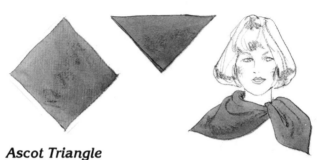

Ascot Triangle
Fold corner to corner to form a triangle. Tie ends for a casual look.

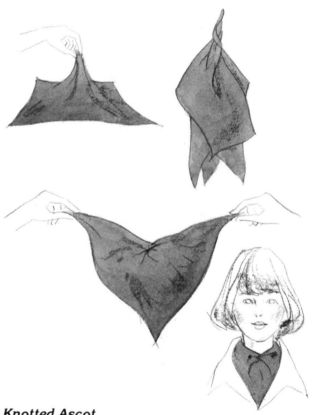

Knotted Ascot
Create an instant Dicky (blouse substitute) by tying a tiny, loose knot in the center of a large, square scarf. Holding opposite corners, fold the scarf with the knot on the inside. Tie behind the neck. Arrange the scarf to resemble a cowl neck blouse under a suit jacket or V-neck sweater.

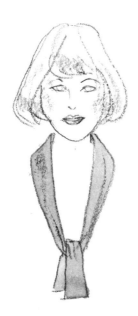

Shawl

Place a long scarf around your neck and tie a simple fold over at the most becoming length to improve the line of jewel necks, boat necks and sweaters.

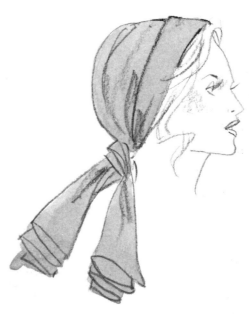

Head Band

To hold a head band or head scarf in place or add height to your scarf, first fasten a strip of foam (available in craft shops) in place with bobby pins. A head scarf tied over the foam strip will never slip.

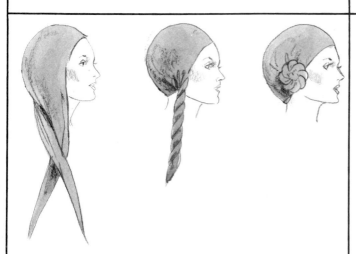

Rosette

The rosette works best with a long chiffon scarf. Simply twist the ends together tightly until the scarf winds itself into the rosette. Secure with straight pins. The rosette also works well on a scarf belt.

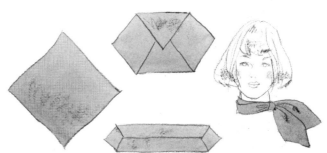

Western Tie

When the corners of your square scarf has pretty designs, fold as shown. If the scarf is large and your neck short, trim off the folded corners and stitch the raw edges together for a less bulky effect.

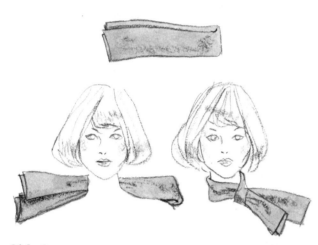

Side Loop

Fold a long scarf crosswise. Put the loose ends through the folded end. Pull snug to the neck. Use straight pin to anchor.

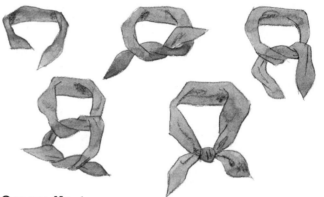

Square Knot

A square knot is a controlled, secure knot, good for scarves or tie belts.

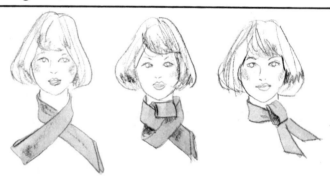

Long Fold-Over

Fold a long, slender scarf in half, crosswise, and tie as shown for a controlled but perky look. A great way to use pins or tie tacks. Try using a pierced-earring as a tie tack.

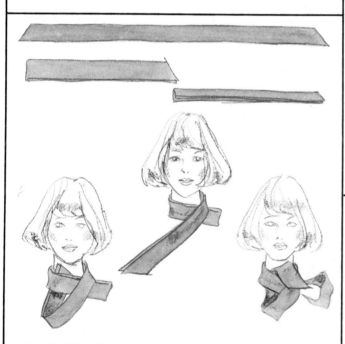

Two-in-Hand

A simple way to achieve a complicated effect. Fold a long scarf lengthwise, then crosswise. Keeping folded end shortest, wrap loose end around neck, loop under, over and through the folded end. Adjust length and pin in place.

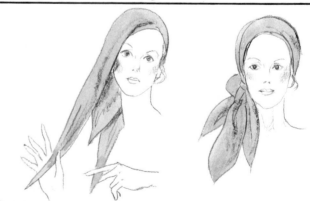

Gypsy

A sophisticated look, especially good under a straw hat for summer wear.

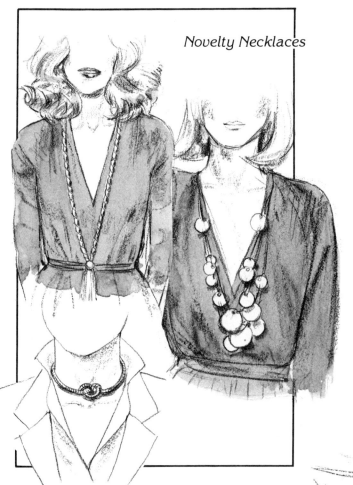

Novelty Necklaces

is gold, you could wear two white-gold ring guards to tie in your silver jewelry or vice versa. Try mixing your gold and silver chains and bracelets.

A simple loop earring in shiny or brushed metal is most basic. For those with small-boned facial features, the smaller the circumference the thicker the earring can be. The larger the circumference the thinner it should be. The larger the facial features, the thicker and larger the earring can be.

A stay-put earring is best. Dangling earrings are for evening or for costume fun wear.

Rings are fun. They should be scaled to the size of your hand, appropriate for the occasion and worn on a well-groomed hand. Movement and noise in jewelry are for daytime or casual wear. Jewelry for dressy occasions should sparkle silently. Jewelry on a public speaker should be motionless. Wear only two pieces of matched jewelry at one time. Unmatched but cleverly combined jewelry is very chic. Combine several necklaces, bracelets or rings.

Jewelry

There are more mistakes made in selecting jewelry than in any other accessory. Costume jewelry runs in bewildering cycles with something new to trap us every year. In choosing jewelry consider whether the outfit is casual or dressy. Scale jewelry to your size. Smaller girls with smaller bones and facial features look better in daintier jewelry. Taller women with larger bone structure and facial features can wear more massive jewelry and more pieces. Winters and Summers wear silver, platinum or white gold. Springs and Autumns wear yellow gold. If you have good jewelry in the wrong color, you could add a few pieces of the opposite metal and wear them together. For example, if your wedding ring

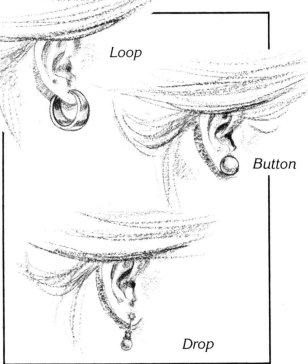

Loop

Button

Drop

METALS, PEARLS AND OTHER MATERIALS

□ Brushed metal is the dressiest, especially if it is used with stones or pearls.

□ Shiny metal is better for sport or casual wear.

□ If shiny and brushed metal are combined, the look will be less dressy.

□ Every woman should own a string of pearls. Real pearls are desirable, but good costume pearls will do. Pearls go anyplace and never go out of style. Winters wear fresh-water white or gray. Summers wear a rose hue. Springs and Autumns wear a yellow hue (cream color).

The texture and weight of your jewelry should compliment the texture and weight of the fabric in your garment.

□ Plastic or ceramic jewelry and shells, seeds, wood, leather, macrame, etc. are casual and should be worn on natural, cotton-type fabrics.

□ Rhinestones and crystal are worn after five. Soft-colored stones may be worn before five.

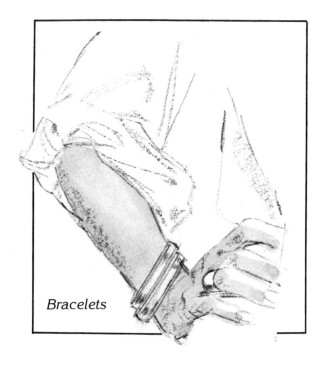

Bracelets

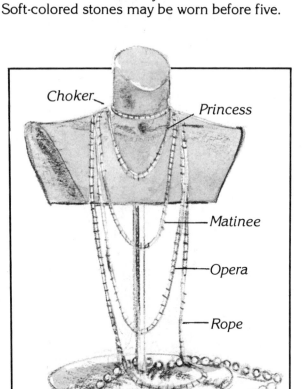

Choker

Princess

Matinee

Opera

Rope

LENGTHS FOR PEARLS OR CHAINS — This

is not a length in inches. You must measure your body to determine the appropriate length.

□ A *choker* fits above the hollow of the throat and looks best on a longer neck. If the neck is thick, wear it looser.

□ The *princess* length falls about halfway between the choker and the matinee. It is the most common length. It is worn on the skin in the open neck of blouses or on sweaters.

□ *Matinee* comes to about the crown of the bust. This is the most versatile length.

□ *Opera length* comes to the midriff. It looks better on a medium to tall, well-balanced figure.

□ A *rope* reaches past the waist. It looks better on a tall girl with a balanced figure.

Graduated beads are not good for narrow shoulders or a full bust because they draw the eye to their center, and then down.

If your dress or suit is intended as the center of interest, play down your accessories. If your garment is simple, add flair. We feel most of our students are underdressed.

Accessories For All Seasons

WINTER — *Fragrance* — Sophisticated, exotic, oriental or spicy scents. Your body chemistry affects the scent. Your perfumes and deodorants should be rotated.

Jewelry — Silver, white gold, platinum, antique silver. Genuine precious stones: diamond, emerald, ruby, sapphire, black opal, crystal, zircon. Fresh-water pearls, white or gray tone. Jewelry should be significant to enhance your strong Winter colors. Scale jewelry to your size.

Furs — Harmonize fur to hair color. Lavish fur of distinct color, either white, gray, dark brown, black or a combination.

Flowers — Camelias, carnations, roses or violets for your lapel. A Winter usually prefers a bouquet or potted plant of poinsettias, azaleas, chrysanthemums, roses or lilies to a corsage.

Woods — Oak, walnut, gray or dark mahogany, cherry, ebony, antique woods.

SUMMER — *Fragrance* — Single florals or floral-bouquet scents: carnation, lilac, gardenia, etc. A pure rose fragrance is delightful.

Jewelry — Silver, white gold, platinum, rose gold. Pearls with a pink hue are best. Stones that have a soft luster: opal, moonstone, amethyst, rose quartz, pink sapphire, garnet, blue turquoise, tourmaline, zircon, aquamarine. Ivory-carved cameo. Jewelry should be simple, modest and smart.

Furs — Harmonize fur to hair color. Gray-brown tone fur or silver mink for gray hair. Summer usually doesn't care for furs.

Flowers — Roses, primroses, azaleas, gardenias, carnations, violets or sweetpeas.

Woods — Ash, maple, walnut, rosewood, mahogany or wood finished in antique white.

SPRING — *Fragrance* — Light and fresh. A light floral fragrance or a combination of spring blossoms: lilies-of-the-valley, violet, lilac, rose or apple blossoms. All flowers of springtime scent. Fruity fragrances. Never heavy or spicy.

Jewelry — Yellow gold, bronze. Stones that sparkle: diamond, aquamarine, zircon, tourmaline, yellow sapphire, topaz, light smoky topaz, amethyst; also coral and opal. Pearls should be ivory with a golden hue, dainty to medium size. Floral ceramic jewelry. One or more lightweight chains. Spring should never have a heavy, bulky effect.

Furs — Harmonize fur to hair color. Off-white to golden-brown fur tones. Gray when hair is gray.

Flowers — Daisies, daffodils, carnations, roses, lilies-of-the-valley, baby's breath, narcissus, blue violets, baby rosebuds. A bouquet of mixed spring flowers is typical.

Woods — Pine, fruitwood, light maple, pecan, teak, oak or walnut.

AUTUMN — *Fragrance* — Mixture of woodland scents and spices. Your body chemistry affects the scents. Your perfume and deodorant should be rotated.

Jewelry — Yellow gold, bronze, copper, antique gold. Best stones are jade, amber, agate, topaz, smoky topaz, opal, onyx, smoky quartz, coral. Pearls should be ivory with a golden hue. Jewelry should not be too dainty. A plain or hand-crafted look is better. Scale jewelry to size.

Furs — Harmonize fur to hair tones. Red to sable brown, gray furs when hair turns gray.

Flowers — Yellow daisies, chrysanthemums, asters, marigolds, zinnias, red poppies, wheat, straw flowers.

Woods — Pine, pecan, teak, maple, oak, walnut, cherry, redwood, mahogany.

Good accessories will elevate your whole wardrobe from mundane to marvelous. Collecting good accessories takes time, discipline and determination. Persist in your search. Accessories provide the finishing touch to your new image.

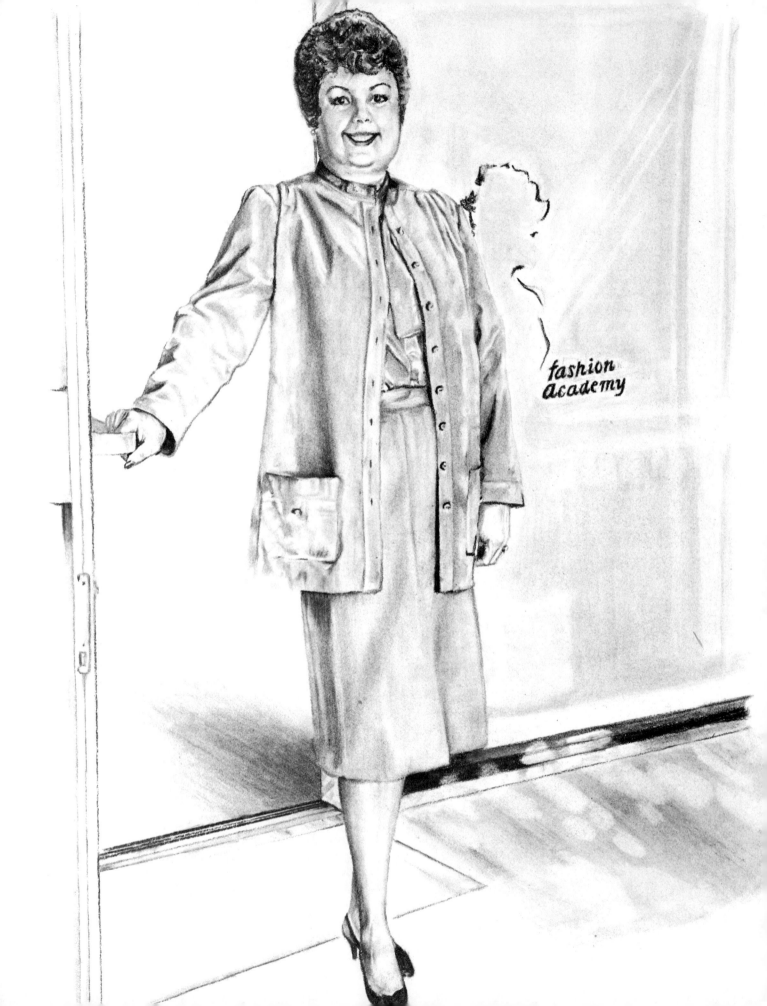

CHAPTER ELEVEN

Potpourri

THINGS YOU NEED TO KNOW BUT HATE TO ASK

This would be a dull world if we were all slender and stately. While most of us like to imagine ourselves ten to twenty pounds thinner, the thought of sacrificing comfort, disposition and favorite foods discourages us from achieving that elusive goal. We would never suggest that everyone should be thin, but we do insist that if you are going to be overweight, you should be the best looking fat lady in town! Looking good requires good nutrition, well-toned muscles and glowing skin.

We do offer a gentle reminder that a five-pound weight loss will make all your clothes look better. A ten-pound weight loss will put you into a smaller size.

We live in a diet crazy era. Every few months some new miracle method breaks upon a gullible world, promising to make us thin and beautiful without discipline or excessive effort on our part. Some of these diets might work for awhile, and if they include all the basic nutrients, they may be harmless. But while experimenting with one diet after another, we are ignoring the hard, cruel facts of modern life. The point is, the only way most of us will ever achieve and maintain a sensible weight level is to re-educate ourselves to the basic needs of the human body, retrain our appetites and expand our lifestyle.

In our years of close association with thousands of students, we have heard about every kind of diet, every crazy method, club, drug, herb or surgical procedure which has flashed across our overweight nation. We have noted that the women who lost weight and kept it off had all come to the same conclusion. We also noted that the rest of the ladies didn't necessarily want to hear about these simple, inexpensive discoveries. They preferred flitting from one diet to another, continually searching for the magic formula that would work for them — effortlessly. Others looked within themselves for deep psychological reasons for their constant battle of the bulge. We maintain that the culprits are very ordinary: sugar, additives, preservatives, affluence, a demand for easy preparation, and fast-paced lives, requiring food to match. We eat too much of the wrong kinds of food and we live largely sedentary lives. Find a regimen which will work for you, one you can live with for the rest of your life, and accept principles that are self-evident:

☐ Eliminate refined carbohydrates. Stop or drastically reduce eating sugar in any form. Because sugar is hidden in most packaged and fast foods, you will have to do more preparing of your own food from scratch or locate specialty stores that offer such sugar-free foods. White flour, white rice or any other food which has been refined (what a terrible misnomer) or over processed, should be left out, or once again reduced, in your diet. This includes some dry cereals, many frozen and most convenience foods.

☐ Eat fresh vegetables, raw whenever possible.

☐ Eat fresh fruit in moderation. We tend to feel so virtuous eating fruit that we overdo it.

☐ Reduce your consumption of meat to a bare minimum. Many of the most successful weight controllers that we know of eliminate red meat entirely. Substitute more fish and fowl for red meat.

□ Eat whole grains, raw nuts, seeds and beans.

□ Avoid carbonated drinks of any kind. Substitute for that can of chemicals a glass of ice water, spiked with fresh lemon or lime — delightful! Cut out coffee. Replace it with the decaffeinated brands or herb teas. Alcohol, loaded with empty calories, is an enemy to your face and your figure.

□ Eliminate most salt consumption. Allow your taste buds to become reacquainted with the natural taste of foods.

□ Remember that small women don't eat much!

□ Accept the fact that you might have a metabolism which can be maintained on very little food. A bright side to this thought is the realization that if there is ever a famine, you will be the last to die.

□ Exercise! The human body cries out for activity. Regular vigorous exercise will result in reduced hunger, better muscle tone and improved skin coloring. Try a variety of exercises until you find some activity you enjoy and one that fits your schedule. The first indications of old age are slow movement and poor posture. Exercise of any kind will help you maintain good body alignment and alert, youthful movement. After all, you are as young as you feel.

TIPS FOR A WEIGHTY LADY — Some of our most beautiful clients are large women. If you are as large as life and want to realize your potential for looking good, you must exert a little more effort.

A good brassiere is an absolute necessity. Choose one with a broad band in back to avoid the bulge resulting from a narrow back band. The construction of the bra must be such that the weight of the breasts is supported by the bra cup, not the shoulder straps. You must have separation of your breasts in front with a defined cleavage. Good cleavage is best attained with an underwire bra. Underwire bras are very comfortable if they are properly fitted. Find a well-informed fitter in a well-stocked store. Keep your bras clean and in good repair.

Good separation or cleavage allows fabric to drape between your breasts — giving a slender front line.

Wear soft, drapey fabric such as lightweight jersey or crepe. Crepe de chine, charmeuse, chiffon or georgette have beautiful drape and will take off pounds. Choose beautiful patterns or designs in your fabric which could not possibly be used for a housecoat or nightgown. Elegant, expensive-looking fabric is worthy of saving and sacrifice.

Tents, floats, and caftan styles of very soft fabric and worn street length will be very becoming. The shift silhouette on the figure with a large waistline, if it is made of soft fabric, will move with the body, giving the illusion of a slim waistline, where there is none. Princess lines are always slimming if they skim the body. Two-piece dresses are a nice change if they are of the shift silhouette.

Don't fall into the trap of wearing your tops too long, hoping to hide a multitude of sins. To the contrary, a too-long top will shorten your legs and make you look heavier and older. Straight, shift-type tunics, street length and sleeveless, worn over a slim-sleeved dress can be the epitome of elegance on the larger woman.

Be immaculate in your grooming. Use deodorant soaps, antiperspirant, perfumes with a light, fresh scent. Manicure your fingernails and your toenails. Wear fresh underwear every day. Don't forget to wash your hosiery after each wearing. Special hosiery detergents can prolong the life of your hose. Find a brand of hose which fits your special proportions in order to avoid a roll above and/or below the waist. If the waistband is too tight, you can loosen it by clipping halfway through the elastic in several places.

Find a hairstylist who is good with your type of hair. Have regular cuts, perms and sets. If you are not skilled in setting your own hair, you can learn to use the new Velcro® hair curlers which require no bobbi pins. Never be seen in public in hair curlers! Also learn to use a curling iron for touch-ups. Beautiful hair will not only make you look wonderful, but will enhance your feeling of self-worth. Find a hair style which is flattering to your face shape and in keeping with your body as a whole. Avoid a too-bouffant hair style which, though it may flatter a full face, will make your body appear heavier than it is.

There is an old adage which says, "If everyone around you has lost their head, but you are calm, cool, and collected — your hair is, no doubt, looking great!"

Learn to apply your makeup with an artful, delicate touch. You have beautiful skin — enhance it with perfectly matched foundation. Emphasize your eyes with subtle rouge and eye makeup.

Wear good shoes. You are hard on shoes, so you must pay for quality. Your shoes must provide support for your feet and control your toes. Avoid thong sandals or any other footwear which might look sloppy. Keep your shoes well-polished and in good repair — especially the heels.

The last tip is a gift from you to your loved ones. You may have become overweight through no fault of your own, perhaps developing poor eating habits during your childhood. Protect your children from overeating. Do not prepare rich or high-calorie foods. Help them learn to enjoy fresh, raw vegetables, fruits and nuts. Do not buy snacks or junk foods. Dump leftover cakes and high-calorie treats into the garbage in the morning, when your determination is high, then no one can eat them in the afternoon — especially you.

FOR TALL, SLENDER GALS — If you are tall and slender, be joyful! Coco Chanel said "It is almost impossible for a woman to be too thin or too rich." Unfortunately, most thin women have lived all their lives around women fighting overweight, and are badly infected with the "try to look thin" disease. Forget form-fitting, shape-defining, revealing clothes — think loose,

blouson, bat-wing, layered, flared, bulk, texture, volume! Collect interesting jewelry, of important dimensions, capable of making a statement. Forget tiny, dainty necklaces, rings, and bracelets which would look cute on your little sister but "cutsie" on you. Get some wide, wild belts and cummerbunds to wear below a bloused top and over a full skirt. You will create the illusion of a tiny waist on a shapely figure.

Don't cut your hair too short. You need enough hair to enable your head to balance your body.

You look marvelous in all the big, stylish fashions your smaller friends would sell their souls to wear — so wear them!

THE SHORT OR STOCKY LADY — The challenge is to appear taller and/or thinner. We are striving for an optical illusion, and the method we use is the same for either figure type.

Keep a balanced hair style, off the shoulders. A large head makes a body appear shorter and fatter. The neck appears longer and slimmer if there is space between hair and shoulders.

Use every possible device to bring the eye to the center: V-necks, center-front detail on clothes, jewelry, buttons, plackets, trim, open collars and narrower lapels. Wear matching tops and skirts or slacks. If the outfit is three-piece, a dark skirt or slacks and jacket with a light blouse brings the eye to the face, and lengthens the body. If the outfit is two-piece, the color of the skirt or pants should be repeated in the blouse, if they do not match.

Flesh tone hose are your best choice. Dark hose which match the hemline and shoe are a fun fad if your legs are slender.

Shoes which match your costume lengthen the line, as do high heels. Even your walking shoes would need to have heels of at least two inches for maximum becomingness. You can even find beach thongs with one-inch heels.

Inset sleeves, vertical seams and applied design contribute to a longer, slimmer look. Depending on the size and balance of your hip, bust and waistline, all silhouettes could be used with the exception of the one-piece drop-waist

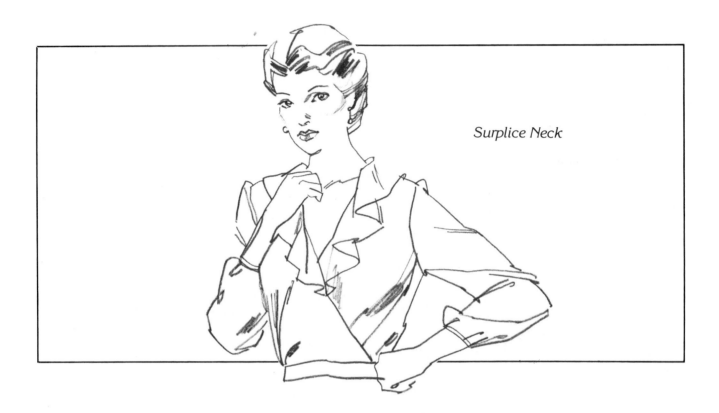

Surplice Neck

silhouette, which would visually shorten your legs. The two-piece drop-waist dress will be excellent, however. (See Chapter 3, page 66.) Jackets with skirts should be no longer than the hipline or break of the leg. Crotch-length jackets should be worn only with slacks. The short woman will look good in hip-line-length jackets with slacks, if her hips are slim. This jacket is most becoming if it is loose at the hip and worn unbuttoned.

FOR A FULL BUST — The most important step is to get yourself into a good brassiere. It should have a wide back band and non-elastic shoulder straps. The weight of the breast must not hang on the shoulder straps. The underwire bra provides the best separation or cleavage. Underwire bras are perfectly comfortable if they are properly fitted.

If you have full, pendulous breasts, grooves in your shoulders and frequent backaches, you are a likely candidate for corrective surgery, which in your case would not be considered purely cosmetic. Most good insurance policies will cover such surgery. Find a plastic surgeon who specializes in breast surgery. Investigate his reputation. This is no time to look for a bargain. There is no type of surgery which does more for the woman who needs it in terms of self-esteem and a sense of well-being than breast reduction. It takes off more years than a face lift.

The trick with a full bust is one of diversion. Divert attention and camouflage the problem with applied design. The primary requirement is for ample bust room in the garment — a question of size. You need to emphasize shoulder width, which will diminish apparent bust size. The device which will best accomplish this is a yoke with gathers over the bust.

Soft fabrics fall gracefully over the bust, and if you have accomplished good cleavage with your bra, you'll look slimmer over the tummy.

V-necks not deep enough to expose too much cleavage are becoming. V-necks with a collar lapel helping to broaden the shoulder are an excellent choice.

Ruffles on a V or a surplice neck are most beautiful on the full bust. The ruffles add a feminine touch and great camouflage.

The full-busted woman will find the Princess silhouette in suits and coats most becoming. The shift is good in very soft fabric if there is good separation between the breasts. The size of your waist and hip will determine whether or not you will belt your shift.

The natural waistline silhouette will be good in a soft fabric. A skirt and blouse in a subtle Crepe de chine print with a short, shaped (Princess) jacket picking up one of the colors of the print is a marvelous suit look for this figure. The raised-waist silhouette is good, particularly in a formal, providing you can get a fit for your full bust.

It is imperative that you have a center interest, V-necklines, jewelry, open collars and lapels. Avoid plain jewel necks and bodices and anything which is too tight.

SMALL BUST — If your bust is small, rejoice! Modern clothes are designed for an "A" cup or "B" cup. Depending on your height, follow suggestions for the tall, slim girl. Use more volume, bulk and texture in your bodice. You can wear bras with fiber fill. We never recommend surgery for breast enlargement, but only you can know how you feel about your flatness. If you are considering implants, do your homework. Find a specialist that does that specific procedure, and check with someone who has had work done by that surgeon. The placement of the implant is critical, a youthful bustline falls just below the level of the underarm.

PROBLEMS — REAL OR IMAGINED — We have attempted to provide guidelines which will lead to a more beautiful you. If you have a problem which we seem to have neglected, write to the Fashion Academy Inc., Costa Mesa, Calif. Describe your dilemma and we will try to help.

MATURITY — Life begins at 40, the fun begins at 50, and contentment arrives at 60! Being 60 is wonderful! It would be even better if we could enjoy the maturity, the status, the control of our lives without the vague aches and proliferating wrinkles. You've bravely met every challenge in your life thus far, however — this is no time to surrender. To help you realize your potential for beauty, we have included some specific suggestions.

Be extremely strict about wearing only your own colors. With maturity, your skin has become more faded and your eyes and hair have lightened a little. You cannot cheat with your colors anymore, even if you got away with cheating when you were younger. Choose your softer, lighter shades, especially near your face.

Wear soft fabics. You may have been a Gamin or a Natural all your life, but now you have earned some ruffles, drapes and gathers. Remember, ruffles come in all shapes and personalities — from softest frou-frou to tiny, orderly little pleats. Dull-textured fabrics flatter your skin, as do feathers and fur. Shiny fabrics compete with your skin and hair, and at this age, who needs the competition?

The petite mature woman has had particular problems. If she ever found ready-to-wear to match her diminutive dimensions, the clothes were more suitable for her granddaughter.

There is, at last, a breakthrough. Petite clothes are available which are well designed and come close to fitting. Manufacturers have still not grasped the fact, however, that the mature woman has a slightly thickened waistline and often a small roll on the upper hip and tummy, which call for a few soft gathers instead of darts. You might want to be sure there is ample seam allowance on the waistband of skirts if you need to enlarge the waist a little. The petite mature woman must beware of "cutsie" clothes. It is time for an elegant Classic look.

Regardless of how thin the mature woman might be, her skin has softened, Very deep "V" necks and exposed midriffs or shoulders are a dead giveaway of your age. Wear sleeves which cover your elbows whenever possible. Small collars or ruffles camouflage a crepey neck.

Mature women need more makeup, but a softer touch and shade. Get a *triple* magnifying mirror, so you can see any makeup goofs or stray hairs which appear mysteriously at a certain age. Following application of foundation and rouge, apply translucent face powder around your mouth with a soft brush, brushing gently to remove excess. Apply your lipstick after the powder. Lipstick will not then "bleed," that is, creep up those tiny wrinkles around your mouth. Avoid frosted makeup of any kind. A shiny look emphasizes wrinkles. A matte finish is more elegant.

If you can learn to apply them, false eyelashes work wonders on mature faces. If you can manage the strip lashes, you will find the individual clumps much easier to apply and wear. Purchase only *short* lashes. The others are ridiculously long and too obviously fake. If your hair or lashes are black, use black lashes; otherwise, use brown.

If your hair style has been sophisticated and smart, it is time to try for pretty. Soft curls around the face soften any lines.

Lighten the color if you dye your hair. You might seriously consider letting the gray show, but only if you are ready for it.

If you hate what the years have done to your face, consider plastic surgery. Do your homework and read a few books on the subject. Your library will have several. Get the names of at least two doctors who specialize in the specific type of surgery you are considering. Spend the money for an examination and interview. No one can tell how you should feel about your face. Whether or not to consider plastic surgery is a decision you should probably make alone. Eye tucks produce miraculous improvement. The eye tuck is an office procedure, and heals in about three weeks. Everything is relative. Many types of plastic surgery cost about the same as the depreciation on a new car for one year.

The mature woman who is satisfied with herself and contented with her progress in life accepts the passing years with equanimity. Most of us have some notion of the lady we would like someday to be — we need to start becoming that lady by age sixteen. Qualities such as tolerance, understanding, wisdom and love don't just happen — they are earned.

Things We Thought Everyone Knew

When putting on your pantyhose, extend, or point, your heel, not your toe. This avoids too tight a stretch over your toes. Your hosiery will wear longer and your toes will be less cramped. It is possible, if your feet hurt, that your hose are tight, rather than your shoes.

Clip your toenails every week. Run a nail file over the ends of your big toenails to smooth the edges. You will have fewer runs. Many of our students freeze their pantyhose to extend wear. Just pop the package into the freezer overnight.

Many perfumes and colognes have dye added for color, which can spell disaster for silk clothes or white underwear. With this in mind, spraying your cologne onto your pantyhose in the hip area will avoid stains. If you want more fragrance near your face, spray a cotton ball with your fragrance, and tuck it into the cleavage of your bra.

If you polish new shoes before you wear them the first time, they will be better able to resist nicks and scratches. When pointed toes on shoes return to fashion, a tiny metal tap applied near the tip of the toe will prevent wear.

Placing a piece of tissue between the lips after applying lipstick will avoid lipstick marks on clothing when you pull them on over your head.

Curl your eyelashes before applying mascara, rather than after, in order to avoid breaking your lashes.

If you are allergic to deodorants or antiperspirants, try taking chlorophyl tablets — available from your druggist. Be prepared for a seasonal green excretion.

When you wear white clothing, undergarments of a neutral color work best. White under white shows every line. Never wear bikini underpants under slacks or if your outer garment touches your hips. The lumps they create look dreadful.

Always remove your garments from the plastic cleaning bags immediately. Clothes are better stored in a cloth garment bag to prevent mildew and to avoid the acid content of the plastic bags. Use plastic, wooden, or best of all, padded hangers. Suits and knitted garments demand padded hangers.

If you use a dipilatory creme or wax your upper lip, do it before bedtime rather than just prior to an important engagement. The skin will have a chance to lose its redness by the next morning.

If you must pull a garment on over your head after your hair has been combed, place a silk or chiffon scarf lightly over your head, tieing it loosely under your chin. Then the garment may be pulled over your head without disturbing your hairdo.

To help tame unruly eyebrows, spray a little hair spray into the palm of your hand, rub it into your brow brush, and brush the brows lightly, after applying your eyebrow pencil.

A Parting Word

Finding your colors, conquering your figure problems, learning to dress in harmony with your personality and defining your lifestyle will enable you to look your very best. The major advantage of looking your best is that when you know you look good, you feel more confident and secure. Spend enough time on yourself each day to accomplish your goal. You can then devote the rest of your time and full attention to others. A woman who is sincerely interested in other people has charm, and that is our ultimate aim for you as you develop your *"New Image."*

Index

FASHION ACADEMY INC.

MODELS — All models in our photographs are students of the Fashion Academy, associates or members of our staff. Each student in the "before" photos was chosen from our classes on the first day of a session. One week later, following an appointment with the staff at Mr. Zachary's Hair Design, she returned to the Academy. Proper makeup was applied, she was clothed in her proper color, and the "after" shots were taken. No professional models were used.

List of models:

Susan Samuelian
Cindi Swenson
Dayna Tanaka
Sharon Murray
Elise Jardine
Ann Hall
Mary Anne Pinckney
Carole Pickup
Pat Fitzpatrick
Sunny Lockie
Nancy Whitlock
Staci Shaw
Terra Anders
Linda Davis
Anya Anthony

Sheri Pinckney-Childress
Emelyn Castleton
Carolyn Yates
Sondra Meith
Cecelia Gomez
Janelle Swenson
Deborah White
Wendy Graf
Naomi Reinertson
April Ricks
Lisa Eddy
Roselyn Spencer
Suzan Brownfield
Sue Porterfield
Joie Green